the crucial years

the crucial years

The Essential Guide to
Mental Health and Modern Puberty
in Middle Childhood (Ages 6–12)

Dr. Sheryl Gonzalez Ziegler

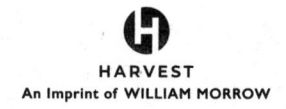

HARVEST
An Imprint of WILLIAM MORROW

This book contains advice and information relating to health care. It should be used to supplement rather than replace the advice of your doctor or another trained health professional. If you know or suspect you have a health problem, it is recommended that you seek your physician's advice before embarking on any medical program or treatment. All efforts have been made to ensure the accuracy of the information contained in this book as of the date of publication. This publisher and the author disclaim liability for any medical outcomes that may occur as a result of applying the methods in this book.

Names and identifying details of some of the people portrayed in this book have been changed.

THE CRUCIAL YEARS. Copyright © 2025 by Dr. Sheryl Ziegler. All rights reserved. Printed in the United States of America. No part of this book may be used or reproduced in any manner whatsoever without written permission except in the case of brief quotations embodied in critical articles and reviews. For information, address HarperCollins Publishers, 195 Broadway, New York, NY 10007.

HarperCollins books may be purchased for educational, business, or sales promotional use. For information, please email the Special Markets Department at SPsales@harpercollins.com.

FIRST EDITION

Designed by Renata DiBiase

Illustrations by Rich Hennemann

Library of Congress Cataloging-in-Publication Data has been applied for.

ISBN 978-0-06-337865-0

25 26 27 28 29 LBC 5 4 3 2 1

This book is dedicated to the girls and their parents who have taken my puberty classes, as well as to Gen Z, Gen Alpha, and the future generations of all kids who need to be seen, heard, and understood.

And of course, for my three kids, Isa, Hazen, and Hudson, may you understand that mental health *is* health, and may you always take good care of it.

Contents

Author's Note ... ix

Introduction: Why Are These the Crucial Years? ... 1

Part I: Understanding Middle Childhood

Chapter 1   Middle Childhood and the Role of Parents ... 19

Chapter 2   The New Rules of Puberty ... 45

Part II: The Foundation of a Healthy Relationship

Chapter 3   The Unexpected Ups and Downs of Middle Childhood: What Parents Can Do to Help ... 87

Chapter 4   The Unexpected Emotional Ups and Downs of Middle Childhood: What Kids Can Do ... 116

Chapter 5   Pressure: School, Social, Sports ... 139

Chapter 6   Understanding Sexual and Gender Identity Development ... 164

Part III: The Tough Stuff

Chapter 7 Body Image and Relationship with Food   191

Chapter 8 Preteens and Success: Shaping Healthier Digital Habits   231

Chapter 9 Substances   270

Epilogue   286

Acknowledgments   289

Notes   293

Index   299

Author's Note

I have been on the front lines of youth mental health for over two decades. As a result, I see and hear about things that may be outside of your or your child's current experiences. My intention is to provide information that I think any parent or caregiver needs to navigate raising children today. Some of it may apply to you and your child, and some may not. If I put it in this book, I feel there is a good chance this issue will impact you or your family in some way, some day. I also believe that knowledge is power. In that spirit, the book is intended to be read in its entirety, but if you wish to skip a topic that's fine too. It will be here if you ever find yourself needing it in the future. While the stories included in this book are about children and families from a variety of backgrounds and circumstances, I've done my best to provide you with research, data, and my own experiences that I think are universal. And last, due to the nature of some of the chapters, please know that triggering topics such as puberty, depression, suicide, anxiety, and body image issues are discussed throughout the book. If you are particularly sensitive to these topics, you may want to take a break from reading, giving yourself some time to process how you're feeling, or, if possible, find someone to help you talk it through.

INTRODUCTION

Why Are These the Crucial Years?

> Encourage and support your kids because children are apt to live up to what you believe of them.
>
> —Lady Bird Johnson

As a clinical child psychologist, I often receive phone calls from frustrated, mystified parents who tell me that their little kids have suddenly morphed into bigger children who they don't seem to understand anymore. One of these calls came from a mother, Holly, whose eight-year-old daughter, Nora, had become highly emotional. For the past few months, Holly told me, Nora would cry at just about anything. Nothing Holly tried was helping, because Nora couldn't tell her why these things upset her so much. Feeling increasingly more frustrated, Holly made an appointment with me.

Sure enough, Nora's deep brown eyes got watery almost as soon as our first session started, and she started tugging on her ponytail. When I asked her what her tears were saying, she whispered fearfully that she didn't know. I assured her we would figure it out together.

Nora is not alone. Every day in my private practice I work with children who are struggling in some way or another with anxiety, friendships, or sudden changes in their emotions or behavior. These kids are in the age group that psychologists call middle childhood—they are six to twelve years old. Many parents are surprised to hear just how formative these years are. There's a lot of cultural focus on the preschool years, the preteen years, and the high school years, but middle childhood has been largely overlooked—that's a problem, because it turns out these years are crucial years, for kids and parents. During this period, children go from losing their first baby tooth at around age six to losing their last tooth at around age twelve. At age six, children leave kindergarten behind them, beginning their formal education. They start to participate in organized sports and other activities, spending most of the day away from parents, meeting new people and forming new friendships. Parents, in turn, start to put more emphasis on academic achievement and extracurricular activities, but may not always have a strong grasp on how to guide a child socially and emotionally.

To add to this already unique phase in a child's life, there's a new, complicated factor at work: the earlier onset of puberty. It's not at all uncommon for pediatric mental health providers such as myself to now treat third and fourth graders who have strong emotions like Nora, who are also starting to develop breast buds or pubic hair, and who almost act like stereotypical teenagers. Girls are starting puberty about a year younger than they did in the 1970s on average, usually between ages eight and thirteen. Boys, who have historically been a year or so behind girls, now start puberty between nine and fourteen. One 2020 study revealed that the age of onset of puberty has actually dropped three months per decade since 1980. The reason for this phenomenon isn't completely clear, but environmental toxins, obesity, and increased stress seem to be playing a significant role in puberty's earlier appearance. Whatever the root cause, there's no doubt that the age at which children enter adolescence (characterized by significant physical, psychological, and social changes as individuals undergo puberty) has been steadily trending downward for decades. So, if you have ever heard someone say, "my kid is nine going on nineteen," there's some truth to that.

When adults hear the words "moody," "awkward," "angry," "confused," "clumsy," and "defiant," most of them think of a middle schooler, maybe age eleven or twelve, who is making the transition from tween to teen. They don't usually think of an eight-year-old. No one Nora knew owned a bra or used deodorant, and she wasn't scheduled to learn about sexual development in school until fifth grade, which was still two years away. But as I explained to Holly, pubertal changes start *in the brain*, not the body, and moodiness like Nora's can be a telltale sign that puberty is on the horizon.

As it turned out, being on the cusp of puberty was only one part of the picture for Nora. In our sessions, this eight-year-old girl—who was an intelligent, curious, and somewhat introverted kid—revealed to me a myriad of issues that were causing her anxiety, including her fears, not just about the usual friendship issues, but about the active shooter drills at her school, and how she would react if there really was a shooting. She shared how sad she was when her teacher taught her that the ice caps were melting and affecting the polar bears' ability to hunt, and how worried she was about the safety of her grandparents who lived in Florida where they were experiencing more hurricanes and flooding. Nora didn't know how to understand or process her very real and valid fears, and her mom didn't know how to talk about them in a way that was helpful given her young age.

In addition to earlier puberty, kids today are bombarded by stressors and technology that neither you nor I encountered and probably could not have imagined when we were growing up: social media, mass shootings, climate change, the long tail of the pandemic, the opioid crisis, and on and on. These children are coming into their own during a time when schools have become battlegrounds over which books should be available and whose version of history should be taught. Kids are figuring out who they are in a time that offers much broader spectrums for sexual and gender identities, identities that you might not fully understand.

Most kids need guidance working through these complex issues, and parents often aren't informed or aware enough to help. Your kids are more aware of politics than you realize. They're more conscious of body image. Although much of the news about the youth mental health crisis has focused on teens, elementary school kids are caught up in the rising tide of psychological issues that threaten to overwhelm America's young people. Unlike Nora, Holly grew up in the 1990s, a relatively more benign time. She didn't have quick and easy access to the internet as a child, didn't have social media, and didn't carry a cell phone; this was the age of a shared family computer and dial-up connection. Holly didn't enter puberty until she was in middle school. Academic and athletic pressures were far less intense. Holly's parents didn't have to deal with escalating college costs and club sports were barely getting started. At Nora's age, Holly hadn't yet heard of climate change and the Columbine High School shooting hadn't happened. Something like 9/11 was unthinkable, as was a global pandemic. People generally believed in science, schools were not hotbeds of politics, and sexuality and gender were presented as more black-and-white. Holly explained to me that, growing up, she thought the world felt fairly safe, and she was not particularly concerned about her future.

In our one-on-one sessions, Holly confessed she was struggling to wrap her head around what was happening with Nora. She kept telling me, "I thought I had more time before I had to deal with teen moodiness!" I told her what I tell all parents with children in this age group—that I want them to flip the switch from experiencing a confidence crisis to *seeing opportunity*.

The middle childhood years are often described as "the forgotten years," but as I tell my clients, this is a crucial time for children—and for parents too. Middle childhood is a beautiful window of time and opportunity to connect with your child and help them build the support structure they need to thrive through the elementary school years and into adolescence. Studies show that parents can actually have the most influence on a child *before* and through the age of twelve.[1] *After* the age of twelve, peers take on a much greater influence in children's lives. In other words, when children are in middle childhood, you can still influence how they think, feel, and behave. You are still the most important model for the choices they make, and the values they hold. During these crucial years, children will still listen to you, they expect to be guided by you, and they still like being around you. You are likely their favorite person in the world. When the teenage years kick in, kids are focused on claiming their independence and figuring out their identity by spending time with friends, leaving little space to be guided by parents in the way they had been when they were younger.

Over a period of months, I worked with Holly and Nora to come up with strategies and tools to better manage Nora's emotions, putting her on a path to a healthier, less fraught adolescence. This wasn't just treatment, it was prevention: I was effectively educating this mother and child on what's to come and how to talk about it, arming them with tools, so that when the predictable issues of adolescence came up, they would both be better prepared.

With some knowledge and education about the middle childhood years, I believe we can *all* put our children on a healthier path, effectively putting the brakes on the escalating numbers of youth with mental health issues that we're seeing across the country and around the world. This is why I've called this book *The Crucial Years*: between the ages of six to twelve you have your widest window to influence the course of your child's future. We cannot wait until the teen years to address the variety of factors that lead to mental health issues. How you parent now can help prevent concerns like low self-esteem, lying, and poor body image. By arming children with effective strategies at an earlier stage, we are paving the way for them to navigate the challenges of puberty and adolescence with resilience, equipping them with the tools necessary for mental and physical well-being. This work is an investment. You are setting the foundation for a more stable and healthier teen and adult life.

I say all of this not to scare you, but to empower you. We can all rise to meet the challenge of supporting kids in today's more complex world. It's not easy to be a kid today in a body that's changing in surprising ways, with a brain that hasn't caught up yet, and won't for years to come. You can help your child thrive today *and* tomorrow.

The following chapters will explain what's happening to your child now and prepare you for what's to come when your tween transitions to a teen. I'll discuss how to talk about puberty, how to help children manage emotions and deal with issues such as gender, sexuality, body image, bullying, screens, and school pressure. You may feel as if children aged six to twelve are too young to deal with these topics, but even if you're not talking about it, they are likely already hearing about these things from peers or online.

Each of the chapters in this book will look at these topics in the context of middle childhood, mental health, and the important competencies your child is developing at this unappreciated, but crucial stage. I'm writing this book because every family can benefit from a better understanding of middle childhood—and I want this to be your essential guide to these years.

WE NEED A PARADIGM SHIFT

A "paradigm shift" is a fundamental change in approach or underlying assumption. Each chapter in this book will include what I see as today's predominant point of view and where I think parents need to shift to stay up-to-date with today's world. Here's the first one:

Paradigm: My child is still a little kid. It's way too early to start talking to him or her about puberty, anxiety, and other issues. Why should I introduce these ideas into their head when they are still so young and puberty is so far away?

> **Shift:** The years from six to twelve, commonly known as middle childhood, can no longer be "forgotten" years during which parents sail between the challenges of early childhood and the turbulence of adolescence. A lot is going on during these middle years, and knowing what to expect and how to best support your child can influence their health positively, now, during the teen years, and into adult life.

My Middle Childhood Years

Writing this book has led me to reflect on my own middle childhood years and the tremendous transitions I went through during that time. I was raised by my immigrant single mom who was still in her early twenties when I turned six. She'd emigrated on a Freedom Flight from Cuba when she was in middle childhood herself, at only twelve years old. A few years later, she met my biological father, an immigrant from Puerto Rico and a Vietnam War veteran suffering from PTSD. They became pregnant with me, and when I was three, they got married and then divorced soon after, so I ended up living alone with my mom between Washington Heights and the South Bronx.

Once I started at PS 98, I ate free breakfast and lunch at the school where I spent kindergarten and first grade. After school, we relied on food stamps, and I went to medical clinics when I was sick that took kids that had no insurance. I only spoke Spanish as I was surrounded by other immigrant families. I didn't have my own bedroom, but I was happy to sleep with my mom or cousins in their beds or on couches. I was "easy." I was "smart." I was identified in kindergarten by Mrs. Wolff (we never forget our teachers' names, do we?) as special. The story goes that she told my mom that she needed to get me out of our situation, that I showed intelligence and something different she needed to nurture. I have profound gratitude for that teacher and for my mom for listening.

At the age of eight my mom married a New York City police officer who was a single father of four in upstate New York, and we moved to an environment that was much less diverse, but where I was happy to have my own bedroom. When I started second grade at my new elementary school, I quickly worked on my English, doing my best to get rid of my heavy accent. I remember playing hopscotch; I remember the girls skipping rope and me teaching them double Dutch. I remember my friends and their families that took me in and treated me so well. I remember my teachers and working so hard to assimilate. I didn't want to stand out. I wanted to fit in, be "normal" and play. I started playing the flute when I was ten, I did my best at school, and I started running competitively and cheerleading by fourth grade. It's amazing to me that in a six-year span from ages six to twelve, so many memorable things happened. By sharing my story here, I invite you to reflect on your own childhood. What was your home life like? Did you move around? If you had siblings what were your relationships like with them? What did you do for fun? Who was your best friend? How did you feel about school?

Today, I'm a clinical pediatric psychologist and I've been working in the field of children's mental health for the past two decades. At my group private practice in Denver, Colorado, I see kids and teens of all ages, while also hosting a regular Start with the Talk class for girls and their parents about puberty and what this means for their physical, emotional, and social growth. As well as being a nationally recognized speaker on the issue of children's mental health, I have a teenage daughter in high school, a son in middle school, and a son in elementary school. I've been living this book as I've been researching it, creating the guide to this age group that I wish had been around when my oldest went through this stage. It is steeped in research but delivered by someone who is both an expert and a fellow traveler. Through my training, research, and own parenting journey, I've come to a deep understanding of the often-confusing terrain of middle childhood. And here's the good news: I've seen the enormous benefits for children *and* their parents when they have the guidance and insight they need to find their way through this period in a child's life.

UNDERSTANDING MIDDLE CHILDHOOD

As I shared earlier, the middle childhood years are often referred to as the "forgotten years" because experts, researchers, and public health advocates have placed so much focus on infancy, early childhood, and adolescence. Think about the parenting books you've come across. Have you ever seen one specifically about middle childhood? Plug the term "middle childhood" into the National Institutes of Health's research database, PubMed, and you get fewer than 2,800 results. Do the same with infancy, and you get almost 74,000 results. Adolescence brings up a whopping 2,350,000 results.

The middle childhood years of six to twelve are like many "middle" things in our society—think middle children, middle age, middle names—often overshadowed by what's on either side. We have common names for children in all the other stages of their eighteen years of development: newborns, infants, toddlers, preschoolers, tweens, and teens. But what about when we get to kids six to twelve? What do we call them? Some people use the terms elementary schoolers or school-age kids; sometimes we call kids on the upper end of this range preteens or tweens. But there is no one term for six- to twelve-year-olds that corresponds to toddler or teen.

I learned years ago that most parents are not familiar with the concept of middle childhood. I remember a mom had asked me how much empathy her child should have at age eight, and when I breezily began, "Well, in middle childhood . . . ," she immediately stopped me. What was middle childhood, she asked, and why had she never heard of it? I realized she wasn't alone. Now, I take more care to explain what developmental phases are, what middle childhood is, and why it's so helpful to understand what to expect during this overlooked span of a child's life.

Here's the lowdown: a developmental phase is a period of growth and change marked by physical, cognitive, and social-emotional milestones. Generally, the agreed-upon developmental stages of childhood are infancy and toddlerhood (birth to age three), early childhood (three to six), middle childhood (six to twelve), and adolescence (twelve to eighteen). (I say generally because these numbers are slightly different depending on which researcher or organization is outlining the stages.)

Why has there been so much focus on early childhood and adolescence? One theory is that it's because these stages have such significant and noticeable changes and milestones, whereas growth patterns take longer and are slower in middle childhood. Another is that once children enter formal education, parents' (and society's) attention often shifts from naptime and potty training to academic performance and achievement. And, finally, parents simply spend less time with their children, who are more involved in school, with friends, and participating in structured activities while parents sometimes feel like they are getting time back for themselves to focus on work or other priorities.

While my focus is on the middle childhood years, my intended reach is much broader than that: this book is your guide to prepare your child for mentally and physically healthier teen years. The teenagers I work with are scrolling on social media, self-diagnosing themselves with mental health conditions like OCD and SAD, using a slew of terms like "toxic," "narcissistic," and "phobic." Yet despite efforts in some school districts to teach them to identify and label their feelings, these teens still struggle to describe anything beyond happy, mad, and sad. Some get taught mindfulness but don't really know how to apply it in real-world situations. The emphasis is on making discomfort go away, instead of seeing discomfort as the signal to pay attention to uncomfortable feelings. Instead of avoiding discomfort, they need to learn to sit with their feelings and understand that they come and go in waves (a lesson some of us are still learning well into adulthood).

The Global Youth Mental Health Crisis

Until the 1980s, most experts didn't think that prepubescent children could suffer from depression, and adolescent sadness was often dismissed as part of typical teenage moodiness. But research has demonstrated that not just teens, but children, too, can experience depression, and that depression among kids is on the rise.

The pandemic opened our eyes to this growing crisis. As researchers measured its impact on kids' mental health, the results were alarming; for example, a study found that mental health–related emergency room visits between April and October 2020 had increased 24 percent for kids aged five to eleven, and 31 percent for those age twelve to eighteen. A Centers for Disease Control (CDC) survey conducted from January to June 2021 found that 37 percent of high school students reported they experienced poor mental health during the COVID-19 pandemic, and 44 percent reported they persistently felt sad or hopeless during the previous year.

In October 2021, the American Academy of Pediatrics (AAP), American Academy of Child and Adolescent Psychiatry, and Children's Hospital Association jointly declared a national state of emergency in child and adolescent mental health. In December 2021, US Surgeon General Vivek Murthy issued a public health advisory, saying that "the challenges today's generation of young people face are unprecedented and uniquely hard to navigate. And the effect these challenges have had on their mental health is devastating."

Both statements noted that this youth mental health crisis wasn't created by the pandemic, although the pandemic exacerbated it. In fact, some experts believe that it might take a generation to recover from the damage the pandemic caused when it robbed young people of important developmental milestones and formative experiences. When researchers looked at the years immediately preceding the pandemic, they discovered that rates of anxiety and depression were already rising.

In 2022, the Employee Benefit Research Institute released a study of mental health and substance abuse insurance claims between 2013 and 2020. It found that of the six age groups included in the study, spending on mental health and substance abuse for children eighteen and younger increased the most, from 12 percent of total health care spending in 2013 to 18 percent in 2020, a 55 percent increase. The CDC also released a report in 2022 that examined data from 2013 to 2019 and found that in the ten years leading up to the pandemic, feelings of persistent sadness and hopelessness increased by about 40 percent among young people.

There are some parents who question whether the reports of the current youth mental health crisis are a product of children simply experiencing the typical growing pains and normal angst of childhood while under a microscope, resulting in excessive and premature diagnoses. It's a good question, and the answer by and large is "No, this crisis is not exaggerated, it's real." I want you to know I have carefully reviewed the data I share with you in this book and I have reflected on my own experiences of treating children over the years. In my experiences, those of my colleagues, and the interns that I supervise—people who are treating kids and teens every day—we can tell you that kids in middle childhood are not immune from the youth mental health crisis. Sadly, I see children in middle childhood who are having panic attacks and the kinds of stress-related gastrointestinal issues I used to associate with teenagers, but who also have tantrums like much younger children. I've had kids as young as six tell me they are sad and they want to die, or that no one would care if they weren't around. The CDC reported that, after declining from 2000 to 2007, the suicide rate for children aged ten to fourteen nearly tripled from 2007 to 2017.

I could base my entire practice solely on treating kids this age who suffer from anxiety. Kids can be anxious about nearly any aspect of their lives: attending school, academic pressures, athletic performance, friendships, bullying, the weather, their health, and more. Anxiety seems to be cropping up in younger and younger kids, like the nine-year-old who talked to me about the overturning of *Roe v. Wade* and wanted to know what she could do about the future of women's rights. Or the handful of kids who come in at the start of the summer with fears of high winds and tornadoes. Young as they are, these children are already thinking they might not marry or have children because they won't have enough money to raise them. They express uncertainty about God, which may be linked to the dramatic decline in attendance at religious services at a time when they need help making sense of the world. During the height of the pandemic, a twelve-year-old, whom I only treated over telehealth video, asked me: "If there is a God, why would he let my grandpa die from the coronavirus?" The number of kids excessively worrying today is staggering. A survey of more than 130,000 kids ages nine to eighteen conducted by the Boys & Girls Clubs of America found that 71 percent say when something important goes wrong in their life, they can't stop worrying about it.

Meanwhile, we don't have nearly enough mental health practitioners to help these children. Between 2016 and 2020, according to a report in the *Journal of the American Medical Association* (*JAMA*), there were increases in anxiety and depression among kids ages three to seventeen, but there was no corresponding increase in availability of mental health treatment or counseling. The AAP described the situation starkly: "Mental health disorders affect one in five children; however, the majority of affected children do not receive appropriate services, leading to adverse adult outcomes."

There are many barriers to treatment for mental health disorders in children: cost, stigma, and shortages of therapists, including bilingual and culturally competent providers. But the greatest is simply a lack of mental health treatment providers. In my own group practice of clinicians, the waiting list was nearly a year during the pandemic and is still months long. When I look for colleagues to refer to, many say they have stopped accepting new patients.

There is a notable shortage in child psychologists. It is estimated that to meet the current demand, an additional eight thousand psychologists are needed. This shortfall is problematic in both rural and urban areas where the supply of psychologists is significantly lower compared to metropolitan areas. Similarly, we are facing a shortage of between 14,280 and 31,109 psychiatrists, and more than half of US counties lack a single psychiatrist.[2] This shortage is exacerbated by the fact that over 60 percent of practicing psychiatrists are fifty-five or older, many likely nearing retirement. More than 150 million people live in areas that are federally designated mental health professional shortage areas.[3]

And the shortage of mental health providers for children is only projected to get worse. The American Academy of Child and Adolescent Psychiatry reported in 2022 that there was only a national average of fourteen child and adolescent psychiatrists per one hundred thousand children, and that the providers' average age was fifty-two. According to data from the American Psychological Association (APA), only four thousand out of more than a hundred thousand US clinical psychologists work with children and adolescents. In 2016, researchers at the Cleveland Clinic and Villanova University predicted that there would be a shortage of almost two hundred thousand social workers by 2030; current assessments think that scenario might now be too conservative.

Meanwhile, ERs are turning into de facto stabilizing centers for adolescents with suicidal thoughts who lack health care. *JAMA* published a report in May 2023 that found that from 2011 to 2020, emergency department visits among children, adolescents, and young adults for mental health reasons approximately doubled. The sharpest increase for the reason for these visits was for suicidal ideation or attempts. Suicide is one of the top three causes of death in children and young adults ages eleven to twenty-four and is a top ten cause of death in five- to nine-year-olds.[4]

According to a 2019 report in the *Journal of Pediatrics*, pediatricians are currently the only source of care for more than one-third of children with mental health problems. But many pediatricians are not routinely inquiring and/or screening for mental health issues. In a 2013 survey conducted by the AAP, 65 percent of pediatricians said they lacked the training necessary to treat mental health problems, 40 percent said they lacked the ability to diagnose mental health problems, and more than 50 percent said they lacked confidence in their ability to treat these patients. These problems are only compounded when you factor in culturally competent care for Black youth who are at the highest risk for suicide attempts and death by suicide. High school students who identify as LGBTQ+ are at highest risk for depression and suicidal thoughts, yet most physicians working in an ER are not trained to treat these adolescents.

However, given the state of the health-care system, pediatricians treat children with mental health disorders anyway, because they have to. It is common for me to meet a new patient who has been diagnosed and prescribed medication at their pediatrician's office, especially for ADHD. Pediatricians tell me they offer basic screening and prescribe medication because they see so many patients with attention issues, depression, and anxiety who would otherwise face monthslong waits to get into a psychiatrist. And while pediatricians usually do refer them to a child psychologist and/or psychiatrist for ongoing treatment, we essentially have doctors on the front line of mental health treatment with little to no formal training. Medication prescribed by a doctor in response to a child's distress may not be the most appropriate treatment; many times the root of a child's issue can be addressed through therapy and parental support alone.

Why You, as a Parent, Are So Important

I say all of this not to be alarmist, but to emphasize the essential role you have as a parent. We're facing an unprecedented global youth mental health crisis with shockingly inadequate numbers of clinicians to treat children at younger ages than before. This is why parents must join the front line. The reality is stark: our children are not entirely all right. But there is something we can do about this.

Everything I share in this book will address one of the three overlapping focuses: middle childhood, puberty, and mental health. My knowledge of these issues is grounded in research and my clinical work and is reflected in my own parenting experiences as well. My goal is not just to enlighten you, but to provide you with practical strategies that will help you prepare your child for adolescence in a way that builds a foundation for a mentally healthy lifetime.

This book is for *every* parent or caregiver of a child approaching puberty, no matter where you live, no matter your racial or ethnic background, no matter your level of formal education. Our kids deserve this. From big cities to small towns, from the White, Black, or Brown experience, from traditional families to nontraditional families, and from binary to nonbinary genders, this book is for you. While I will refer to "boys" and "girls," because that is what most of the research, as well as my experience, is based upon, I also devote a chapter in this book to gender and sexual identity development. I have chosen to alternate the pronouns "he" and "she" in the chapters, but almost all of my guidance is applicable across genders. I will also be referring to "parents" a lot. But let me be clear that this book is for anyone who is a part of children's lives: parents, teachers, educators, grandparents, aunts and uncles, coaches, leaders, nannies, and volunteers.

Each chapter in this book is organized around a paradigm shift, a way of reframing how we think about this phase in a child's life. I will then tell you *why* we need to shift our thinking about the issue, and *how* we can shift our response. You can dip in and out of chapters, based on your concerns, but I would really encourage you to begin with the first section of the book, which explains the overlap between earlier puberty and middle childhood, and offers some very foundational parenting concepts and strategies.

When I say that parents need to learn some strategies for handling these issues, I'm by no means suggesting you need to be your child's therapist or you can head off every potential mental health problem. I know you are likely experiencing your own insecurities: you're bombarded with bad news about the world and your children's ability to handle it; you don't know where to turn for help because, often, help isn't readily available; and you may not feel equipped. But with the right tools, you can set your child on the right footing, for adolescence and beyond. After all, you already have a parenting tool kit for things like teaching your kid to ride a bike or kick a ball, or for dealing with scraped knees and high fevers. You just need to add some mental health–related tools to teach your children how to cope with the complications of puberty and to be able to recognize the signs of depression, anxiety, low self-esteem, and even disordered eating, so you can get your kids help should they ever need it. The good news is that once you become aware of the signs and symptoms to look out, you can become equipped with skills that can help your children through this transition in a way that leaves them stronger and better prepared.

I'm here to serve as your guide, ready to offer concrete solutions to the questions lingering in your mind. I am also here to shine a light on common issues that you may not even be thinking about. I will be sharing real stories from two decades in practice, stories where I've carefully altered identifying details to safeguard privacy. These narratives reveal experiences that might resonate with you or your child, unveiling the shared challenges many have faced alone. In addition to sharing anecdotes, I offer a psychological road map for the journey your child is about to embark on, crossing the bridge to adolescence.

Many things have changed about childhood since you were in elementary and middle school, but some things have stayed the same. Kids in middle childhood are still under construction. They are forming their worldview; they are figuring out what they are good at and where they belong. They are trying out independence, yet they need you as much as ever. At age six, your child may still believe in Santa Claus and the Tooth Fairy. By age twelve most children have grown out of these beliefs—a sign of your dwindling influence on the structure of their minds' imaginations.

As the parent of a child between the ages of six to twelve, I want to remind you that your job is the long, joyful, and challenging process of raising an adult. Your child at this age is learning to feel secure enough to do things for herself, before she transitions to the greater independence and responsibilities of adolescence and young adulthood. Right now, you are your child's manager, in charge of almost everything in her life. Eventually you will retire from your manager role and become a consultant—a role that, if all goes well, you will have for a lifetime.

Whenever you can, slow down and appreciate this precious time. Between the ages of six and twelve, kids are downright delightful, retaining their childish sense of innocence and wonder. They are inquisitive, carefree, and very often funny. They idolize their teachers, adore their parents, and are willing to express love and affection. They'll even still hold hands with you! An elementary school teacher once told me that one of the reasons she loves kids in middle childhood is that they are going through so many firsts: first school bus ride, first time performing in a play, first book read, first show-and-tell, first ball in the hoop, first science experiment, and so on. Unlike the teenage years, when they will often hide their excitement for fear of being uncool, kids at this age are open and full of possibility. The world is still their playground! Middle childhood itself is a special time, even if it's a complicated one. *New York Times* science writer Natalie Angier called it an "essential luxury item" in development. I love that description because it reminds us to appreciate the years that evolution has gifted humans at this stage: a period between the rapid and relentless growth periods of early childhood and adolescence in which children can explore, learn, and grow—with you at their side.

PART I

Understanding Middle Childhood

CHAPTER 1

Middle Childhood and the Role of Parents

> It's not our job to toughen our children up to face a cruel and heartless world. It's our job to raise children who will make the world a little less cruel and heartless.
>
> —L. R. Knost

Hannah and Chris were parents who came to my practice concerned about their nine-year-old son, Brandon. They described Brandon as a naturally anxious child who did well academically, but who had always struggled to fit in socially. He was reluctant to try anything new, whether it was new activities, new food, or new friendships. As a result, he didn't have any close friends, preferring to spend time in his comfort zone with his parents and siblings, or playing video games. His parents confessed to me that Brandon was their youngest child, and his two older sisters tended to get more focused attention in the family, with Brandon tagging along to their many activities. The parents described their youngest child as somewhat "difficult," "closed off," and "resistant," but, until now, they had shrugged off his challenges, assuming he would grow out of them. When Brandon's third-grade teacher identified him as having trouble participating in class and finishing his assignments—she believed it was due to anxiety—the parents found their way to me.

In our intake session, I realized that Hannah and Chris were loving parents who wanted to do whatever they could to help Brandon, yet despite having two older children, they had no idea where to start. Brandon's sisters had gone through elementary school without needing any extra support, and these parents were flummoxed by Brandon's inability to do the same. In our intake session, I explained that their son was going through a pivotal developmental phase and that it's very common for children to struggle at this age. I wondered aloud if they knew anything about the milestones of middle childhood. Their answer was an emphatic no. "We thought once he grew out of the toddler years, things would be smooth sailing," Hannah confessed. "Of course, he'll eventually catch up with his siblings," Chris added.

When I ask parents what they know about the developmental phase of middle childhood, like Hannah and Chris, they usually don't know what I am talking about. Contrast this to earlier developmental periods of infancy and the toddler years, when you were on high alert for milestones such as smiling, walking, and talking. Part of the reason you were so aware of your child's developmental stages is that it was pounded into your head that it's important to catch any delays early, so you could do something about them. As it turns out, the same is true for middle childhood.

As the Canadian pediatricians V. Kandice Mah and E. Lee Ford-Jones have written in a paper called "Spotlight on Middle Childhood," "Middle childhood, from six to twelve years of age, is often known as the 'forgotten years' of development because most research is focused on early childhood development or adolescent growth. However, middle childhood is rich in potential for cognitive, social, emotional, and physical advancements."[1] Socially and emotionally, middle childhood is a period when children establish stronger relationships with peers and begin to develop a sense of identity. Friendships become much more important—and complicated. Children start to figure out what they like and don't like, and which peers they really want to spend time with. They become more aware of social norms, values, and expectations and they begin to understand the perspectives of others. Cognitively, children at this stage develop logical thinking, problem-solving skills, and increased attention spans. They acquire more advanced literacy and numeracy skills and start to apply them in academic settings. In other words, there is a lot going on—and a lot that can go awry.

In my experience, third grade—or ages eight to nine—is often the time when developmental lags and deficits begin to show up in children, perhaps due to a combination of increased expectations at school coinciding with the greater complexity of relationships at this age, and the beginning of earlier puberty for some. For many kids, third grade can be one of the most challenging years in elementary school, often catching parents, and even educators, off guard.

In our subsequent sessions, I talked Hannah and Chris through some of the key milestones of middle childhood. This is where parental education is so important. Let's say that your nine-year-old has no close friends, like Brandon. If you don't know that the middle childhood years are an important time for developing peer relationships—and that nine is the age when children's friendships tend to deepen in their complexity—you might not notice if your child is struggling socially, or you might take a wait-and-see approach, thinking it's a phase, as had been the case with Hannah and Chris. If you *are* aware of the importance of peer relationships in middle childhood, however, you can take action. You can begin planning short, structured one-to-one playdates with potential friends or encourage your child to join an after-school club that reflects their interests. In this way, we came up with strategies for Brandon to have greater exposure to social situations with his peers, rather than tagging along with his older siblings' playdates and activities.

I pointed out to Hannah and Chris that taking steps to help their child gain better social skills really matters. A 2011 study of Canadian fifth and sixth graders showed that having a best friend could buffer a negative experience by preventing a rise in the stress hormone cortisol. Another study from 2018 of English students ages seven to eleven found that friendships were especially important for children's feelings of self-worth.[2] And a 2015 study found that the quality of friendships in early adolescence could predict how healthy people are as adults. So, a child who doesn't learn how to make close friends in middle childhood could be at risk for increased stress, lower self-esteem, and even poor health into the teenage years and beyond.

Instead of waiting for Brandon to "grow out of it," Hannah and Chris made his social development much more of a priority. As a result, he shared more at home, socialized more at school, and continued to play more with friends after school. When you have an awareness of the various milestones of middle childhood, you can become more proactive in supporting your child where needed. That's what this chapter is going to help you to do.

> **PARADIGM SHIFT**
>
> **Paradigm:** My child is past the preschool years, he's on an even keel now. He's in school all day, the teacher says he's doing well, he can read and write, and he's involved in the things he likes to do—finally things are settling down and I can have some time for myself.
>
> **Shift:** During middle childhood, your child is going through major cognitive, social, emotional, and physical stages. Now is the time to use your influence to support your child's needs, helping him to find what he's competent in, encouraging his decision-making skills, especially as it pertains to relationships, so he can become more independent, which will ultimately give you time back later.

Why Six to Twelve?

Before we delve further into the developmental stages of middle childhood, we should understand where the idea for it came from.

There is some historical precedent for differentiating between ages zero to five, ages six to twelve, adolescence and young adulthood. In earlier eras, children were assigned responsibilities at ages five to seven, something seen across cultures. Children contributed to the household and had chores like collecting and preparing food, making fires, watching after younger siblings, and washing clothes. When they matured physically through puberty and reached adolescence, this would be celebrated with coming-of-age rituals, often marked in some way: by donning a hijab or turban, by wearing long pants or putting up one's hair, by becoming a bar or bat mitzvah, or by going on a vision quest or walkabout.

Nevertheless, until the 1900s, Western culture mostly viewed children as small adults. Sigmund Freud, the founder of psychoanalysis, was the first to construct a theory of human development and divide childhood by stages. In the early 1900s, he theorized that a child's personality developed during five "psychosexual" phases, including a period from six to twelve that he called "latency."[3] Freud described the latency stage as a period of psychosexual development occurring roughly between the ages of six and puberty. During this stage, Freud believed that the sexual impulses of the phallic stage were repressed and dormant, allowing children to focus on developing social and intellectual skills. Freud thought that the latency stage was crucial for the development of communication skills, self-confidence, and the ability to form relationships. According to this theory, the successful navigation of this stage prepares children for the challenges of adolescence and adulthood by enabling children to channel their energies into productive pursuits. This may have made sense more than a hundred years ago, but the age of puberty has fallen dramatically since then—girls now enter puberty five years earlier than they did in the early 1900s.[4] While modern psychology has largely turned away from Freud's focus on psychosexual stages, which hasn't been backed by research, his belief that the experience of early childhood affects development remains a key contribution to the field of psychology.

Swiss psychologist Jean Piaget was the first to conclude that children thought inherently differently than adults—an insight that laid the foundation of developmental psychology. In the 1930s, he devised the first theory of cognitive development, or how children develop intellectually. He, too, settled on five stages, including one that corresponds to middle childhood. Piaget said that during ages seven to eleven, children go through a "concrete operational stage" in which children improve their problem-solving skills and start to think more logically, although abstract thinking remains a challenge and ongoing process.

After Piaget, the German American psychoanalyst Erik Erikson formulated his own theory. Although influenced by Freud, Erikson focused more on socio-emotional development than psychosexual development and believed that people continued to develop throughout their lifetimes. In this theory, each developmental stage comes with a conflict, and as a result, children either successfully or unsuccessfully resolve that conflict as they mature into the next developmental stage. Erikson, too, has a stage that corresponds to what we think of as middle childhood, age six to eleven, during which the main conflict a child faces is a sense of *industry versus inferiority*. As kids take on new challenges and their social world expands, they begin to compare their accomplishments and abilities to others'. Children in this stage strive to develop a sense of competence and achievement by mastering new skills and tasks, particularly in school and social settings. Successfully completing this stage leads to a sense of industry, where children feel capable and confident in their abilities. The lack of success at this stage results in feelings of inferiority, where children doubt their skills and feel inadequate. The goal is to have children emerge out of middle childhood feeling industrious or self-confident.

We can see that early thinkers in developmental psychology agreed that the period of six to twelve was a distinct stage. And, of course, this idea is reflected in our education system's grouping of ages six through eleven in what is known as elementary school.

Middle Childhood and the Tooth Fairy

For developmental and biological reasons, the period of ages six through twelve coincides with the phase where children are losing their baby teeth. For most kids, losing the first tooth is a cause for joy and celebration! It's not just that the child has lost a tooth, it's that he realizes he's "a big kid now." For parents, this can be a symbolic moment too—your child is no longer a baby, with the loss of the tooth as a physical reminder.

In the years to come, as your big kid loses one tooth after another, he will no doubt delight in finding money or a treat under the pillow from the Tooth Fairy. Most parents have a lot of fun with the Tooth Fairy phase—although as the child loses his fifth or sixth tooth, the Fairy may occasionally forget to place money under the pillow because she's either busy or has forgotten to go to the ATM! And when your child finally loses his last tooth, you may even experience bittersweet feelings of nostalgia that this phase is ending. My own daughter lost her last baby tooth the morning of the day she also got her first period—talk about the end of an era!

Losing baby teeth is reminder that middle childhood follows a clear arc, beginning at six and ending at twelve, and that in the same way your child loses his baby teeth, you will also lose some of your influence over him as he grows. At age six, when your child sheds his first tooth, he will still wholeheartedly buy into the stories of the Tooth Fairy, leprechauns, the Easter Bunny, and Santa Claus. Somewhere along the road of middle childhood, he'll realize that adults have made these figures up, but he will continue to play along for the fun of it. Then, as your child grows into a tween, he will no longer believe in these stories, nor need them. And when he is twelve and thirteen, you will realize you no longer have the same influence you once had to shape the way your child sees the world. And so, every time your child loses a tooth, let it be a reminder that middle childhood is a journey filled with countless gains—and some loss, too. And that in the same way your child is growing adult teeth that will last him a lifetime, the way you nurture him now will stay with him forever.

Ages and Stages in Middle Childhood

When your child was a baby or toddler, you probably had a clear idea of the different milestones to expect, like sitting, standing, and walking. Now that your child is progressing through middle childhood, he's still going through major developmental changes; you're just less likely to be aware of what they are and how best to support them. To help you have a better understanding, I've listed the major changes you can expect to see year by year. I want to make clear that all children move at their own pace and your child doesn't need to check every single one of these boxes to be considered "normal." Instead, I want you to use this list of social-emotional descriptions to set healthy, age-appropriate expectations for you and your child, so you can give him additional support if needed.

AGE SIX

Social-Emotional

Your six-year-old is interested in making friends. He will usually engage in imaginative play, and while cooperative play may start now, he may still struggle with sharing and taking turns. You can expect him to engage for a limited amount of time in small-group activities. He will become more and more aware of social norms and expectations and will practice emotional intelligence and empathy by showing care and compassion for others. He might do this by kissing a boo-boo or getting a friend a Band-Aid. His conversations will typically be focused on what is happening in the moment, and he will be able to identify emotions such as happy, mad, sad, scared, and excited within himself and others.

Self-Esteem

He may start to value his worth in terms of distinct areas called "competencies," such as how he learns, how he dances, how he builds things. He isn't yet comparing his abilities to others.

Problem-Solving

At this age your child uses play to figure things out. He is less likely to demonstrate aggression toward peers as a way of ending disputes, but he likely still needs the help of an adult to solve social problems.

Moral Development

He is still in the formative stage of determining what is right and wrong, fair and just, and is oriented toward fixed rules. He will often rely on his immediate family's rules as a guide in the world.

Self-Expression

Kids this age also use imaginative play to express what they have been experiencing and processing. Allowing for free, unstructured play is a way to facilitate self-expression at this age. At this age, your child can usually verbally state whether they are happy, mad, or sad. He is also aware that certain body or facial gestures express feelings.

Responsibility

He is typically eager to help around the house and spend time with his parents and can do such things as putting away his own toys, pulling weeds, and wiping down the table after a meal.

Attention Span

Attention span is generally calculated to be two to three minutes per year of age, so twelve to eighteen minutes of sustained attention can be expected at this age.

AGE SEVEN

Social-Emotional

This is when kids start developing closer friendships. Your child will begin to recognize his own strengths and weaknesses, and to understand how to apply social norms and rules in different situations. He is better able to identify and label a limited spectrum of feelings and start engaging in teamwork in sports and on the playground.

Self-Esteem

He is ready to try new things and set small, measurable, and reasonable goals for himself and engage in positive self-talk.

Problem-Solving

Solving problems starts to occur in groups and may still be challenging for him.

Moral Development

He begins to understand and differentiate between right and wrong and demonstrate a growing awareness of fairness and justice.

Self-Expression

He'll likely enjoy art, talking more, writing or doodling in a journal, singing, dancing, or playing music. It's normal to have a variety of interests that may come and go at this age.

Responsibility

He's ready to do things like take care of his own personal hygiene, feed pets, and water plants.

Attention Span

About fourteen to twenty-one minutes.

AGE EIGHT

Social-Emotional

He begins to form deeper friendships and consider other people's perspectives. He can understand the concepts of reciprocity, taking turns and compromising. He starts to pick up on jokes, sarcasm, and social cues. His conversation becomes more detailed and expressive, and he is better at processing his thoughts and feelings. He may identify as belonging to a certain peer group.

Self-Esteem

He seeks increased independence and starts to form a clearer sense of self. He wants to be liked and validated and seeks approval from peers and adults.

Problem-Solving

He becomes better at working with peers to achieve common goals in games and activities and resolving conflicts through communication and compromise.

Moral Development

Children are generally respectful of rules and authority figures at this age and understand their role in maintaining order and fairness.

Self-Expression

He enjoys joining in group activities, clubs, and team sports, which can provide opportunities to identify with peers who are like-minded.

Responsibility

He can dress independently, prepare his own backpack for school, complete homework independently, and sort laundry.

Attention Span

Sixteen to twenty-four minutes.

AGE NINE

Social-Emotional

Friendships get more complex, and he may have a few close friends he prefers to be with. Interest in social media is piqued. They pick up on social cues and nuance and start to understand more complex emotions, such as pride, guilt, shame, and jealousy. Disappointment and frustration are still difficult to handle, but progress is usually observable. This age is particularly complex for girls, who start to experience "drama," and mean-girl behaviors may begin.

Self-Esteem

He begins to compare himself, his family, and material objects to others, wanting to fit in and be as good as—or better than—others. He responds especially well to positive feedback and praise.

Problem-Solving

He can solve many social problems independently and begin to use strategies regarding conflicts such as pausing to take a deep breath or talking to a trusted adult, although not consistently.

Moral Development

He becomes more compassionate and willing to help others, understanding his role in contributing to order or chaos and what his values are. This age is the beginning of separating from what their parents' morals and expectations are to shifting to his own.

Self-Expression

He starts to focus on specific interests and may express viewpoints that differ from those of his family.

Responsibility

He starts to become interested in taking on advanced responsibilities, such as making his own lunch, asking for help from adults outside of the family when needed, and helping bring in and put away groceries.

Attention Span

Eighteen to twenty-seven minutes.

AGE TEN

Social-Emotional

Friendships continue to get more complex and by now bullying or hurt feelings may have affected your child's social life. He starts to understand the nuance of social hierarchies and peer pressure may become more of a factor. Differences in physical development due to puberty beginning may cause confusion. He becomes better at emotional self-regulation and at taking no for an answer, turning to sports or art activities to relieve stress. He understands the concept of mixed feelings.

Self-Esteem

He can typically state his own strengths and weaknesses and accept them. His self-esteem is influenced by a combination of peer relationships, personal achievements, and perceived failures. Positive feedback from peers and adults contributes to a healthy self-perception. Girls are likely to be well into the physical and emotional changes of puberty, which can affect self-esteem.

Problem-Solving

Negotiating skills improve and he may choose to confide in or rely on friends for advice on problems, rather than parents.

Moral Development

He may begin to anticipate and ask for help navigating moral dilemmas. He typically becomes more concerned about others and has a well-established sense of conscience, experiencing feelings of guilt or remorse when he believes he's acted inappropriately, often without having to be told. He can understand the reasons behind rules.

Self-Expression

He may start journaling; creating videos; or writing stories, raps, music, or poems to express his thoughts and feelings. He may start posting on social media. Listening to music he likes may begin at this age, as does more interest in clothing, jewelry, and hairstyles—whether or not his parents approve of his choices.

Responsibilities

He can get himself fully ready for school and out the door, do simple yardwork, and take care of personal belongings such as charging a laptop for school.

Attention Span

Twenty to thirty minutes.

AGES ELEVEN AND TWELVE

Social-Emotional

The start of middle school may find him initially sticking with old friends yet also wanting to make new ones. He is likely to be experiencing or be surrounded by others going through a lot of changes and moodiness, but he still processes his feelings openly with family if the norm for doing so is already established.

Self-Esteem

Gender differences in confidence become striking at this age. While boys tend to develop perseverance, determination, and leadership, girls tend to form self-doubt, be less likely to raise their hand in class, and can become pleasers. Girls' self-esteem starts to dip at this age where they become self-conscious of their weight, body type, and overall physical appearance. Boys may become self-conscious about their bodies too as they start puberty at different rates and comparisons around physical growth can begin.

Problem-Solving

He starts to analyze risk-taking, and an increase in attention span may help by allowing him to test out solutions.

Moral Development

He begins to understand that there are consequences to his actions and will usually seek counsel from parents on moral or ethical dilemmas.

Self-Expression

Girls tend to be more verbal and express a wider range of emotions at this age than boys. Boys tend to express themselves through their interests. Both boys and girls may be more comfortable expressing themselves in ways that may be different from perceived norms or what others want them to do.

Responsibilities

He can bring in mail, take out and bring in trash cans, do household tasks such as vacuuming floors, dusting, and cleaning off countertops.

Attention Span

Twenty-two to thirty-three minutes.

The Stages of Active Parenting

Parents develop alongside their children, something I learned from the work of Ellen Galinsky, a researcher who studies child development and family dynamics. Just as your child is developing, so are you. I've conceptualized my own four stages of parenting development based on child development, with each stage being unique and requiring different skills and knowledge, so you have some context for your role in middle childhood and beyond.

Children Ages Zero to Six: Discovery Parenthood

The skills parents develop revolve around physical care, health and safety, discipline, and boundary setting, as well as attachment, love, and nurturance. It's rapid, and change seems to happen nearly every month; parents often report this time to be the most physically taxing as it takes a toll on sleep, routine, and the life they knew before they had kids.

Children Ages Six to Twelve: Exploration Parenthood

Parents have settled into their new role. They are still learning a lot but typically feel more at ease. Teachers and education play a much more significant role in a child's life, and parents spend a lot more time away from their child. The hours they share are more frenzied: filled with homework, after-school activities, sports, or playdates. Weekends are busier too, though each year builds up to events where they can drop off their child and enjoy some time to themselves, something not as readily available before this stage.

Kids Ages Twelve to Eighteen: Challenging Parenthood

Adolescence is usually a time of challenge and change. A child is likely seeking their own identity through time spent out of the home and with friends. When they're home, they can be quiet, withdrawn, and moody. Parenting a teenager means they suddenly speak a social language that parents no longer understand. A teen may have strong thoughts and opinions about clothes, music, and entertainment that differ from his parents'. The challenge for a parent here is acknowledging a child's independence, negotiating limits, and respecting boundaries. Parents generally describe this time as emotionally draining.

Changes in Middle Childhood

Remember Erikson's developmental theory: a child needs to master the conflict in each developmental stage in order to develop the strong sense of self he will need for a mentally healthy life. If a child masters the social, cognitive, and emotional demands of middle childhood, he will exit that stage feeling competent, which leads to greater self-esteem, better ability to manage conflict, and positive social skills, all of which will serve him well in adolescence and beyond. If he doesn't master these challenges, however, the transition from child into adolescent can be filled with insecurities that affect the next stage of identity versus role confusion.

As I explained to Hannah and Chris, if their son Brandon didn't get the experience of making friends and building up confidence in elementary school, it was going to be a lot harder for him to develop friendships in middle school—at which point he would be too old for his parents to set up playdates for him! I was also concerned Brandon would be unprepared for the pressures of modern adolescence that require kids to be able to do things on their own.[5]

I see this in my practice, and it goes beyond friendship. Kids who didn't learn how to be responsible for their own homework in middle childhood are beaten down by the rigors of high school. Kids who haven't developed empathy struggle to make meaningful connections as teens. Kids who have low self-esteem are at greater risk of being bullied or getting into abusive relationships as they get older.

To be prepared social-emotionally for adolescence, when your child exits this middle childhood stage, he should have:

- Declared some autonomy from his parents
- A positive sense of self, including confidence and perseverance
- Displayed empathy toward others
- Competence in his ability to build new friendships and put effort in schoolwork
- Abilities in teamwork, cooperation, and work ethic

Self-efficacy is a belief in one's own competence and is a central tenet to this stage of development. Lack of self-efficacy leads to low self-esteem, and low self-esteem is linked to mental health challenges in adolescence, such as increases in anxiety and depression.

Developing Competency

One point I need to make in this age of over-involved parenting is that kids need to do the work of building self-efficacy for themselves. If you try to do it for them or prevent your children from taking risks and experiencing failure, you will actually get in the way of the main objective of this stage, just as carrying a baby everywhere would prevent that baby from learning to walk.

Here are some ways I encourage parents to help their children develop competence:

- Include your child in discussions about a variety of topics and issues—such as why chocolate is their favorite ice cream, the pros and cons of having homework over the summer, or the news about the latest wildfire. Encourage them to share their opinions without inserting your own.
- Encourage your child to think independently, especially from his peers. Independent thinking is one of the hallmarks of leadership.
- Prompt your child to set academic, social, and physical goals. For a child in this age range this could be learning how to do division, attend overnight camp, or ski a black diamond. Setting goals means tracking progress, which reinforces effort. Even if your child doesn't fully achieve the goal, he will be able to acknowledge the steps taken toward that goal.
- Challenge your children to imagine the future. Good conversation starters are: "Do you think people will ever live on Mars?" "What is something you would want AI to do for you?" "If you are a parent one day, what is something you won't make your kids do?"
- Recognize your child for well-thought-out decisions and problem-solving. In middle childhood, the part of the brain that deals with decisions is still very much under construction, so you want to strengthen the circuits that led to a good decision by rewarding him with specific praise and reinforcement. This may sound like "I noticed that when your younger sibling was having a fit at the store today, you handed him his favorite toy and made silly faces, which made him smile. Thank you, that really helped calm him down and allow me to finish food shopping." Use this level of detail rather than simply saying, "Good job," which is vague and may not reinforce the specific action you want them to do more of.
- Find the right time to help your child reevaluate poorly made decisions and problem-solving. While it's important to point out what went well, it's equally important to discuss what didn't work out. This may sound like "I noticed today when your sister was having a meltdown at the store,

you got angry and yelled at her and then made fun of her for crying. I wonder what else you could have done to be helpful?" Once he answers, you can assure him he will have another chance to practice that skill.

Puberty overlaps during middle childhood in a way that it hadn't in the past. It's not surprising that when puberty and middle childhood overlap, puberty usually takes precedence in terms of what you may see and react to. Even though your eight-year-old daughter may be developing breast buds and need a bralette, or your nine-year-old son has grown so tall he needs longer pants, keep in mind your child still needs to be guided through the social-emotional milestones of middle childhood. Otherwise, your child could wind up with what is called "asynchronous" or "uneven" development, in which his body is ahead of his brain. (Asynchronous development can also show up the other way in gifted children, who may be ahead cognitively but not socially-emotionally.) The best thing you can do is remind yourself that *emotionally* your child is still his chronological age and treat him as such. Just because he might be taller or more developed physically than some of his peers shouldn't change how he is treated, spoken to, or even held.

Parenting Styles

Now that you have an understanding of what you can expect from your child during these crucial years, you'll need to step in and support him when he needs you. But to do this job effectively, you'll want to be honest with yourself about your parenting style. Who were your models? What patterns are you repeating? Does your partner parent differently?

We all have a natural parenting style that we default to, based on how we grew up, whether we're emulating our own upbringing or reacting against it. As I got to know Hannah and Chris in my sessions, it became clear to me that they came from very different backgrounds and had very different parenting styles. Hannah, by her own admission, was the "good cop" in the partnership, emotionally attuned, empathetic, always there to give hugs or lend an open ear. But she struggled with being an authority with her children, often failing to set boundaries for them, or for herself. When she became overwhelmed, she would often snap at the kids in frustration, and then would feel horrible and guilty for doing so. Chris, by contrast, was the "bad cop"—the one who was clear about boundaries and limits for the kids, but who was often rigid, brushing off or making jokes about any emotional issues his kids had. When his children didn't immediately follow his direction, he would often lose his temper.

In my sessions with Brandon, I learned that he often felt out of control, ping-ponging between the differing expectations of his parents. Before Hannah and Chris could better support Brandon, I needed to get their parenting approaches aligned. "That doesn't mean you both need to parent the exact same way," I explained, "but it does mean you need to find some more middle ground, especially around values and expectations."

If you spend any time reading parenting books or on social media, you might hear about different parenting styles, such as gentle parenting, free-range parenting, helicopter parenting, and lawn mower parents. Then you have the tiger moms and panda parents. Popular parenting styles come and go. As their names imply, they are more metaphorical than based on psychological research.

In my practice, I draw from the work of developmental psychologist Dr. Diana Baumrind, known for her pioneering research on parenting styles. Her work, which began in the 1960s, has had a significant impact on the field of child psychology and parenting studies. Baumrind's research focused on understanding how different parenting styles influence child development and behavior. Dr. Baumrind coined the terms: authoritative, authoritarian, and permissive parenting; researchers following her added uninvolved/neglectful. These four styles, often shown on a matrix in which one dimension is **responsiveness** and the other is **demandingness**, have stood the test of time.

Here's a rundown:

AUTHORITATIVE: HIGH DEMANDINGNESS, HIGH RESPONSIVENESS

This is the sweet spot for parenting. Authoritative parents are supportive and show interest in their kids' activities and lives but are not overbearing; they allow children to make mistakes. They have high expectations and support their child in meeting those expectations. They set firm limits and boundaries while being nurturing and loving. They are parents who encourage open and honest communication and listen to their child's point of view. While they don't always do what their child wants, they are willing to listen. Children whose parents use the authoritative style are generally happy, capable, and successful. They are friendly, energetic, cheerful, self-reliant, self-controlled, curious, cooperative, and achievement-oriented.

Example

Parent: Hey honey, I noticed you didn't finish your homework today. Let's talk about what happened.

Child: I didn't feel like doing it. I was bored after school and wanted to play instead.

Parent: I understand that you were bored and wanted to play. Everyone needs a break after school. However, it's important to balance playtime with responsibilities like homework. Next time, how can we make sure you get your homework done and still have time to play?

Child: Maybe I can get a snack, do my homework right when I get home, and then play after.

Parent: That sounds like a good plan. Let's try that tomorrow and see how it works. If it doesn't work, we can figure out another plan together. Remember, I'm here to help you if you need it. How does that sound?

Child: Okay, I'll try that.

AUTHORITARIAN: HIGH DEMANDINGNESS, LOW RESPONSIVENESS

This type of parent values control, power, obedience, and even fear. Yelling, corporal punishment, and high expectations with little support are common practices in this style of parenting. These parents don't typically see anything wrong with what they are doing. They may believe that fearing a parent is good and that spanking or a "whooping" can be effective ways of teaching kids a lesson. They generally think it is acceptable to answer a child with "Because I said so." It can be difficult to convince someone with this style that it leads to poor outcomes, because sometimes children comply in the short term. However, studies show that kids raised in homes such as these have higher rates of anxiety, depression, and aggression and lower self-esteem. They often have difficulty relating socially, managing their emotions, and thinking independently. They also can struggle with authority figures.

Example

Parent: Hey, I just looked in your backpack. Why didn't you finish your homework today?

Child: I was bored and tired and wanted to play instead.

Parent: That's not okay. You know the rules. You must finish your homework before you do anything else. No more playing until all your homework is done, understand?

Child: But can I just do it after I play, I do work all day long in school . . .

Parent: No. I don't want to hear another word from you. From now on, you will come home and do your homework right away. I don't care whether you are tired or bored, there's no excuse. If you don't finish it, I will take away your iPad for the rest of the week.

Child: Okay . . .

Parent: I expect you to follow the rules of this house. Now, go to your room and finish your homework right now.

PERMISSIVE: LOW DEMANDINGNESS, HIGH RESPONSIVENESS

Permissive parents tend to be very loving and well-intended yet provide few guidelines and rules. If they do provide rules, they often fail to follow through on them or are talked out of them. These parents do not expect mature behavior from their children and often seem more like a friend than an authority figure. Parents like this rarely say no to their kids and use bribes such as candy or toys to get their children to behave. Some of these parents are intellectually aware that things need to change but cannot cope with the emotions of making changes. Children of permissive parents often have challenges in interpersonal relationships as well as higher rates of substance use and mental health issues (especially mood dysregulation). They also can have behavioral problems and come across as spoiled and entitled.

Example

Parent: Hey sweetie, do you have homework to do?

Child: Yes, but I am tired and don't want to do it.

Parent: Oh, well I guess that's okay. I would feel tired too if I was at school all day. Playing is important too. Do you think you might feel like doing it later?

Child: Maybe, but I really don't want to right now.

Parent: That's fine, everyone needs a break once in a while. I can email your teacher or you can. If you need my help, let me know.

Child: Okay.

UNINVOLVED/NEGLECTFUL: LOW DEMANDINGNESS, LOW RESPONSIVENESS

Uninvolved parents, sometimes referred to as neglectful parents, make few to no demands of their children and are often indifferent or dismissive of their child's interests and desires. There is a lack of affection, love, and support. Of all the styles of parenting, these children usually fare the worst. They tend to be drawn into abusive relationships and have very low self-esteem. The one positive outcome that can be borne out of necessity in response to this style is that a child gains resilience and self-sufficiency. However, this depends on several environmental factors, including social support, that may not be present for many of these children. Neglectful parents often had neglectful parents themselves and don't consider the damage they are doing. Parents who know they were raised in neglectful family homes should seek treatment so that they do not pass on generational trauma to their own children.

I doubt many people go around thinking, "I want to be an authoritative parent," and I don't expect you to, either. What I hope you take away from these descriptions of parenting styles are the terms **demanding** and **responsive**. These two words alone can guide your parenting: you need to be demanding (high yet reasonable expectations) and you need to be responsive (show support and praise). Love, attention, affection, and protection may form the foundation of a stable childhood, but how much you expect of a child and how you respond to them will determine how strong the structure built on that foundation becomes as they respond to increasing pressures and stress.

To relate this to the parents you met at the beginning of the chapter: Hannah was a permissive, low-demandingness, high-responsiveness parent, and Chris was an authoritarian, high-demandingness, low-responsiveness parent. In our sessions we worked together on balancing their approaches, so that Hannah could get more in touch with setting expectations and Chris could work on his responsiveness. To give one example, when Brandon got home from school, he was supposed to put his lunch box and water bottle in the kitchen, but he never remembered to do it, which inevitably caused problems the following morning when these items would still be in his backpack and not in the kitchen. Both parents would get annoyed in his or her own way. If Hannah was preparing the lunches, she'd call for Brandon to bring his lunch box and water bottle, he would ignore her, then she would get exasperated, running to get the items for him all the while feeling annoyed that he'd failed to follow a rule. If Chris were making the lunches, and Brandon disappeared upstairs to his room, Chris would start shouting up the stairs, berating Brandon, telling him that he was lazy and forgetful, words that really upset Brandon and made him want to hide under his covers. Once we made it *a clear rule* that every day when Brandon came home from school, he had to bring his lunch box to the kitchen before going up to his room—with both parents committed to checking that it was done—mornings became a lot less stressful, and Brandon felt a sense of competency that he could remember to do this task.

Maintaining clear, consistent expectations for your child isn't always easy. Your child will disappoint you, and you will disappoint them. This part of parenting will require you to be open about your personal history, triggers, strengths, and weaknesses, and to be willing to work on your story of who you are and how you got here as a parent. This is hard work—you *will* find it challenging, especially if you have a complicated family history or are navigating parenting with someone who has a different parenting style. But knowledge is power. Once Brandon's parents had some basic understanding of the middle childhood years—and a greater awareness of expectations and parenting styles—they were able to support Brandon together.

The Importance of Play

As I explained to Hannah and Chris, there was another factor that I felt could help Brandon significantly: time to simply play. As the youngest of three children, his parents were often in a hurry for him to "grow up" and keep up with the pace of his older siblings. As a result, he spent a lot of time racing around from one activity to another. Typically, when children attend school all day, parents often feel the need to enroll their kids in multiple after-school activities, especially when they see that this is what all the other parents are doing. They feel as if children must be busy, productive, and "always learning" in order to keep up or even get ahead.

Free play time should be a priority. During this stage, learning still occurs in play, just as it did when he was a toddler or in preschool. Even if your child says they are bored, trust that this is time to be creative, which is a valuable learning experience.

When parents hold space for children to play, they're giving the gift of time doing something that has no right or wrong way. Play allows children to do something where the outcome is irrelevant, and where they can get absorbed in the moment. My message to all parents with children this age is to allow your kid to get messy, be silly, read easier-level books sometimes, and play with rocks, sticks, and sand. This won't "dumb them down" as one dad once said to me while I was playing puppets with his nine-year-old son. *Encouraging*, not just allowing, unstructured play during the middle childhood years provides children with a much-needed outlet and portal, advancing their cognitive/problem-solving abilities; physical, social, and emotional development; and sense of needed mastery. Reminder: this is the phase of a child's life where gaining a sense of competency is key—so give them opportunities to do that, including through play.

In the world of play therapy, we say that play is a child's language, and the toys are their words. So whether it is a toy or a performance your kid wants to put on for you—just let him! Don't tell your child "You're too old for that now," or question if they really want to play with a certain toy. Brandon benefited from spending time alone building with LEGO, playing Nerf guns with friends, and a round of Uno with his parents.

This time was invaluable to Brandon as it allowed him to practice reading how his friend was feeling, if his friend was bored with the game, or how to change the rules. In these situations, the two of them negotiated what they would do next. Play teaches not only social skills, but other important skills like cooperation, compromise, and creativity.

When you create time to get on your child's level and play with him, I call it "dosing." Just a short amount of quality time goes a long way. It helps you to cherish the joys of this age: the quirks, the laughs, his interests, his chattiness are all things your child wants to share with you. And it helps your child feel more connected and understood by you at a time when they still seek your validation and approval.

Even when your child has a growth spurt and looks older than his age, don't forget to slow down and let him enjoy being a child. When my daughter was eleven, she still played with dolls, buying outfits for them from Goodwill. When my son was ten, he still slept with his "lovey" at night. I know a girl who wore a tiny little braid in her hair all through sixth grade; it was her thing. And there's no more committed Halloween costume designer than an eight- or nine-year-old. Just because your child is starting to look like a mini teenager, it doesn't mean you have to put away the dolls, blocks, and trucks. In fact, you should actively encourage him to continue to create and let off steam in this way for as long as possible.

CHAPTER 2

The New Rules of Puberty

Disgust: Hey, guys? What's pub-er-ty?
Joy: I don't know. It's probably not important.

—Disney Pixar's *Inside Out*

When my patient Ava was eight years old, I noticed that she kept tugging on her shirt in our sessions. When I gently commented on this, she told me, "I don't have any bras yet, and I feel like my 'you know whats' are starting to stick out and it's embarrassing!" Ava was too self-conscious to talk to her mother about this, especially because her parents had never broached the topic of bras or puberty.

When I mentioned this to Ava's mother, Carolyn, in our next parent session, she was surprised and a little upset with herself. "I just thought we had more time," she insisted. "Ava seems so young: and her breast buds have just barely started to show. I didn't think they were big enough to need a bra." I carefully explained that even though Ava was only beginning to develop, she was already self-conscious about how she looked in a T-shirt, uncomfortable during playtime or other activities like sports, not liking how her chest felt when she was running and jumping. "Ava needs a bra so she can continue to be the confident and outgoing girl that she is," I explained.

It makes sense that parents like Carolyn don't feel ready for this new phase in a child's development. With puberty happening at earlier ages, it may feel like you're on unfamiliar ground, especially if you yourself began developing much later. Ava's mother wasn't ready for her daughter to have a bra, but Ava *was* ready. In fact, Ava had taken her mother's silence on this topic to mean she couldn't talk to her mom about it, and so she turned to Google to figure things out. The results left her feeling overwhelmed by all the images of breasts and bras she'd seen.

When I discussed with Carolyn that Ava assumed she couldn't talk to her about this, Carolyn seemed especially rattled. I wondered aloud what her own experience of puberty had been like, and we ended up talking at length about what had been a lonely and confusing time for her. Carolyn explained that at Ava's age, her mother had recently passed away, and, with only her father and two brothers in the house, she felt like she had no one to turn to. She saved up her allowance to buy herself a training bra, and a friend's older sister helped her get pads after she got her period. When she visited friends' houses, she would look through their medicine cabinet trying to figure out whether she needed items such as douches and vaginal anti-itch cream. As she described how alone she had felt during this time, she grew emotional, caught off guard by the memories. Her mother was never far from Carolyn's mind, but having a daughter who was suddenly going through puberty made her think again about her loss and how much she had hidden from her dad.

Women aren't the only people with less-than-ideal puberty memories. My husband's father never talked to him about anything related to reproduction or puberty—he didn't even teach him to shave—and neither did his mother. One of his friend's fathers got *Playboy*, however, and in sixth grade the two boys started looking at it in secret, which generated a mix of excitement and shame. Later, my husband, who was predisposed to fainting spells when he was younger, lost consciousness in seventh-grade sex-ed class, although he still insists the topic of the class had nothing to do with it.

The one thing my husband's father did was hand him a book called *What's Happening to Me?* and say, "Read this." The book gave information that hasn't aged well: it tells boys that if they want to know what other growing penises look like they should look at other boys' penises when they are in the locker room! And it informs girls that they shouldn't worry about their growing and changing breasts because boys find them attractive.

No wonder then, that for many of us, conversations about puberty can feel awkward. In this country we have been socialized not to speak freely about sexual development and bodily functions, and many of you might have gotten more helpful information about deodorant, bras, and tampons from friends or older siblings than you did from your parents. In my sessions, I encourage parents to use appropriate terminology when talking about body changes. Most of the adults in the room tell me that their parents used euphemisms like "pee-pee" for penis and "hoo-hoo" for vagina. This baby talk can make discussing private body parts more comfortable for adults, but kids need to have the appropriate terminology, so they don't get a sense that these body parts are something to be ashamed of and so they can communicate effectively with others about potential medical issues or sexual abuse. Using the correct terminology about their bodies empowers children to set and maintain boundaries. You might have trouble getting buy-in from grandparents (one grandmother I know refers to a vulva as a "volvo"; another calls breasts "pillows"), but if they persist, you can simply tell your child that times have changed since their grandparents were young, which is a concept most kids understand. If you yourself have been using euphemisms—that's okay! You can just start transitioning to the accurate terms by telling them that now that they are getting older, it's time to use the correct names.

As Ava's story shows, it's so important for parents to feel comfortable talking about puberty—often long before you may feel ready—because our children need our guidance more than ever, especially when they're turning to online searches to fill gaps in their knowledge. One thing I've observed, both in my practice and in the puberty talks I give, is how little some parents and professionals know about the physiological and psychological developments of puberty. Part of that lack of knowledge has to do with the message we probably got when we were younger that puberty is embarrassing or even shameful, and a lack of sex ed that left us confused about what was going on in our brains and bodies (let alone those of the opposite sex). So we just muddled through.

But that kind of muddling through isn't working anymore. According to a 2020 National Health Statistics Report from the CDC, the median age for getting a first period decreased from 12.1 years in 1995 to 11.9 years in 2013 to 2017, dropping three months per decade. With kids going into puberty at such young ages, parents need to understand how puberty works, so you can explain these changes to your child in a matter-of-fact way and head off any worry or confusion they might end up feeling. Puberty is a process that involves children's brains and emotions as well as their bodies, and the way you manage it now can have a significant impact on your child down the line.

A note on the terminology I'm using in this chapter: in medical terms, early puberty is known as "precocious puberty," and it's defined as going into puberty under age eight for girls and under age nine for boys—although it's much more common in girls. Some recent studies have even found an increase in precocious puberty during the pandemic, perhaps because of stress and social isolation. But while the numbers may be rising, actual precocious puberty is still rare.

For our purposes, in this chapter I am using the term *earlier* puberty to mean when it occurs *before* middle school, the age that most parents assume puberty will begin. This may happen as young as eight for girls and nine for boys. Parents I meet in my practice are seeing the onset of puberty that they typically associate with teens in their elementary school kids. Combined with the myriad of societal issues kids are facing—such as the impact of screens (which we will discuss more in chapter 8)—it can feel overwhelming for parents and kids alike.

Earlier puberty is often confusing and concerning to parents—especially as no one seems to know exactly why it's happening at increasing rates. Theories as to why this is so prevalent include exposure to environmental toxins that affect hormones, the childhood obesity epidemic, or the impact of stress on growing bodies. Some populations, like young Black girls, seem to be more vulnerable to earlier puberty due to racial and socioeconomic factors. Research suggests that earlier puberty in girls correlates with a disturbing number of poor outcomes compared with starting puberty on time or even late. These outcomes include higher likelihood for depression, anxiety, substance abuse, eating disorders, body dissatisfaction, externalizing behaviors, sexualization of girls, risky sexual behavior, early sexual activity and subsequent increase in pregnancy and abortion, breast cancer, and obesity.[1]

Please don't feel you need to run out and buy organic milk or start hounding your child about her weight in a misguided effort to delay puberty! Earlier puberty is a societal issue, not a problem that parents alone can solve. All the healthy habits I endorse in this book—eating a balanced diet with minimally processed food, getting quality sleep, using strategies to reduce stress—are practices I want all kids to start now to maintain a physically and emotionally healthy life, not necessarily to stave off earlier puberty.

Part of the problem is that we are so far behind in acknowledging this reality of earlier puberty that we don't even have the language to discuss it. What do we call an eight-year-old like Ava who has started developing? She doesn't fit into any of the common categories of preadolescent (usually nine to twelve), tween (also usually nine to twelve), or adolescent, which is such a broad range, defined by the World Health Organization as ages ten to nineteen and referred to as "the stage between childhood and adulthood."

Children in the earlier years of middle childhood aren't equipped for puberty. Their bodies may be maturing faster, but their brains are not: Their prefrontal cortexes, which are responsible for restraint and reason, will continue developing throughout the years of adolescence. This means that kids under the age of twelve aren't ready to understand or process many of the feelings and situations their changing bodies might lead to and won't be for some time. Socially and emotionally, they still have a lot of work to do to transition out of middle childhood successfully. After all, eight-year-olds are still learning what compromise is!

Often puberty isn't even on the radar of your typical eight-year-old or her parents. A 2015 CDC survey found that only 21 percent of elementary schools were educating kids about puberty, and just one in five middle schools teach all the essential sex education topics recommended by the CDC. At the time of writing this book, states such as Kentucky, Indiana, Arkansas, and Florida are passing or considering laws that would ban sex ed and discussion about periods until fourth, fifth, or sixth grade—much too late for what our kids are currently experiencing. Even pediatricians—who are on the front lines of responding to parents' questions and worries—may not be ready for modern puberty. A 2020 survey concluded that "a concerning number" of pediatricians weren't following the recommendation of the AAP regarding educating patients about menstruation and feminine hygiene products and "exhibit knowledge gaps in this area." And, of course, parents aren't ready, because you likely didn't go through puberty at such a young age—and you're likely not being prompted by schools or doctors to prepare your kids. Like Ava's mother, you may want your child to remain a child and to not have to deal with periods, body hair, acne, body odor, and all the other changes that puberty can bring.

But we all need to get ready. Research shows girls and boys, but especially girls, who reach sexual maturity and are able to reproduce at ten or eleven years old are also at higher risk for sexual exploitation, grooming, poor peer choices, and earlier sexual experimentation. According to the 2020 National Health Statistics Report from the CDC, the younger a girl was when she got her first period, the more likely she was to have had sexual intercourse at an earlier age: for example, by age fourteen, 20 percent of girls who had their first period at age ten or under had had sex, compared with 5 percent of those whose had their first period at fourteen or older. While rates of depression among children are roughly equal between girls and boys in middle childhood, in mid-puberty, the ratio becomes two to one girls to boys.

Parents who think their kids are reaching puberty too early often mourn what feels like an end to childhood that has come too soon. They feel as if they are being robbed of time with their little kids. They also worry that their children aren't ready to deal with their own—or their peers'—developing bodies in an era of easy-to-access misinformation online. While these are totally understandable feelings, I find it helps to think of this time as an opportunity to start new—and yes, sometimes uncomfortable—conversations with your child. Many kids are already uncertain or worried about the changes that are happening to them or to their friends, and if they aren't already worried, they may pick up on a parent's own feelings of anxiety and confusion. On the other hand, if you can show your child curiosity and appreciation for this transformation of her body and brain, this will help set a positive tone for the entire transition. Regardless of your child's age, it really is an awe-inspiring process that can be celebrated whether a child is eight or fourteen.

In other words, you, as a parent, have the power to give your child a healthy, smooth transition into puberty by taking shame, embarrassment, and confusion out of the equation. The first step in helping children navigate these years safely is to understand what puberty is and why earlier is the new normal. The goal is to handle your child's development with a lot more openness and understanding than you likely experienced when you were this age. Then, you can begin to have matter-of-fact, straightforward conversations about puberty with your child that can continue as she grows—and I have tips and scripts for you in the chapter to help you on your way. I'll also explain how to help kids adjust to physical developments such as breast growth, body odor, periods, acne, and more, which may be showing up at younger ages than you remember.

PARADIGM SHIFT

Paradigm: Puberty is something that's happening to my elementary school-age child in the future. It's not something I have to worry about yet, and I don't want to upset my child by talking about it now.

Shift: Puberty is happening earlier in children than it ever has before, and many schools do not provide the health ed your child needs in younger grades. Even if your own child doesn't develop early, it's likely that his peers will be showing signs and that there will be a lot of schoolyard talk on this subject. By getting ready for this conversation now, you can help your child navigate this transformation with less embarrassment and greater openness and understanding than you likely experienced as a child.

Sound Familiar?

- It seems like every month your kid's pants are too short, and they are asking for new shoes every other month.
- Your kid is either growing more hair on their arms and legs or the hair on their head is getting oily.
- Slight facial blemishes like little bumps on their face are starting to appear.
- A deepening of your son or daughter's voice has you wondering who is calling your name!
- T-shirts are starting to have sweat stains and socks and shoes are starting to smell.
- You find yourself saying things to your friends like "My kid is eight going on eighteen!"
- All of a sudden your child wants more privacy and is closing their door. They may be styling their hair, listening to music, or staring at themselves in the mirror.

- Stories about crushes, boyfriends, and girlfriends are being talked about in your back seat or on FaceTime with friends.
- Body sprays, deodorant, and styling products are new items on your shopping list for your kid.
- There is a new or heightened interest in looking good, smelling good, and being cool.

FAQ About Puberty

SO WHAT EXACTLY IS PUBERTY?

Puberty is the transitional span of time in which a child's body develops the ability to reproduce. It also kicks off a phase of brain restructuring that can prompt changes in moods, emotions, and thinking patterns, which only seem to exacerbate a child's physical evolution. These changes don't happen all at once, however: puberty can last anywhere from two to five years, and the younger a child is when they start, the longer it takes. Girls begin puberty up to two years earlier than boys.

Think of the brain as the body's command and control center. It signals that it's time for a child to start sexual development by sending hormones throughout the body through the bloodstream to tell certain organs what to do. When the hormones reach their destination, they bind to special receptors in the cells of that organ and relay the orders.

In both boys and girls, the process starts with a part of the brain called the hypothalamus, which dispatches gonadotropin-releasing hormone to the pituitary gland (also in the brain). This triggers the pituitary gland to release two more hormones (luteinizing hormone and follicle-stimulating hormone) and direct them to the testicles or ovaries. In boys, these hormones instruct the testicles to start releasing another hormone, testosterone, which will set off other changes, such as the production of sperm, growth of body hair, the deepening of the voice, and the building of muscles. In girls, these hormones instruct the ovaries to start creating estrogen, which leads to the development of breasts and curves, and eventually the monthly release of eggs and menstruation.

When it comes to body odor, the culprits are the adrenal glands, which sit on top of the kidneys. They have their own maturation process—called adrenarche, which means the awakening of the adrenal gland—which usually occurs slightly before puberty. In adrenarche, the adrenal glands increase their production and release of hormones called androgens, which contribute not just to body odor but to genital and underarm hair growth and increases in oil production that can lead to acne. Researchers assume the brain controls this process, but they are not sure what sets it in motion.

Adrenarche might remind you of another word associated with puberty: "menarche" (the onset of menstruation). There are two other "-arche" words related to puberty: thelarche, the onset of female breast development, and pubarche, the appearance of sexual hair.

WHEN WILL THIS HAPPEN?

Puberty can start as early as second or third grade. For girls, changes start between eight and twelve years of age. For boys, changes typically start between the ages of nine to thirteen.

Bodily maturation can proceed on very different timetables and still be normal. Unless your child is right in the middle of the development spectrum, she is likely to be sensitive about puberty's physical transformations. Also, because many of these changes are in the so-called bathing suit area, you might not be aware of how far along your child is in the process.

WHAT ARE THE FIRST SIGNS AND STAGES OF PUBERTY?

For Girls

For most girls, the first physical change of puberty is breast development. It starts with small, firm, tender lumps (called breast buds) under one or both nipples. The breasts will slowly get larger over the next year or two but may continue to grow for years after the first bud is evident. Soft hair will appear on the outer labia (the folds of skin surrounding the vagina). Later, the hair will grow coarser and cover more of the pubic area and appear under the arms.

A girl's body shape begins to change as her hips widen. Expect her first period to start about two years after breast buds appear, usually between the ages of nine and fifteen. Most girls have a growth spurt about one to two years before their period starts. After they get their period, most females add one to two inches of height before growth stops.

For Boys

For boys, changes start with the testicles getting larger. Long soft hair will appear at the base of the penis, before turning darker and coarser and spreading to other parts of the genitals. The penis will also get larger. Boys will have more frequent erections and might ejaculate in their sleep, aka a wet dream.

As puberty continues, hair will grow under the arms and on a boy's face, usually above the lip at first. A boy's voice will also begin to deepen. While this is happening, their voices will crack at times.

A boy's body shape begins to change as his shoulders broaden and he gains weight and muscle. A growth spurt usually happens between the ages of twelve and fifteen. By age sixteen, most males have stopped growing, but their muscles will continue to develop.

For Girls and Boys—Changes in the Brain

In addition to the physical changes of puberty, we need to factor in the changes that happen not in the body, but in the brain. Most parents don't realize that puberty actually begins in the brain—so your child may start to experience unexpected mood changes and behavioral issues before she shows any physical signs of outward development. The release of pubertal hormones actually triggers a restructuring of the brain, with some areas being pruned and some being strengthened with an increase of neural connections. This can lead your child to have much stronger feelings, and to perhaps act in ways that are confusing or feel "out of character" for her. When this happens, it can help to remind yourself that a major restructuring is going on in her brain right now—and this truly isn't your fault or anyone else's. It's also important to remember that this reshaping presents an opportunity for you. The way that you talk to your child and the way that you can help her understand what's happening, not just in her body but her brain, can have a profound impact.

Your child's interactions with you and the ways that you respond to her can actually affect how her brain is rewired.

HOW DO I EXPLAIN PUBERTY AND REPRODUCTION SO MY KID UNDERSTANDS?

Conversations about puberty can be awkward, and the more awkwardness your child senses in you, the more they will feel that there is something embarrassing and shameful about puberty.

Parents often ask whether the mom (or female) caregiver should talk to a girl and the dad (or male) caregiver should talk to the boy. My response is that while there is typically more comfort for both the parent and the child in such situations, it is not necessary, and in many families, it is not even possible. In fact, I think it's great for both parents (if a child has two parents in their life) to be comfortable talking about these issues. But the reality is that when a mother and father are present, a child may feel more inclined to go to the mom for feminine hygiene products and to the dad for tips on shaving.

With my daughter Isa it was easy and more natural for me to start talking about puberty, getting her period, choosing pads, and picking out her first bra. She even helped make videos for my puberty course. With our second child, Hazen, I bought him a book and then instructed my husband to talk to him. My husband, Steve, looked at me, bewildered, and said, "Aren't you going to do this?" I said that while I could, I thought it should come from him. But the truth was that my spouse wasn't prepared; no one had ever had this type of talk with him. Other than one awkward night, when he flipped through the book with our older son, I've been the one leading the talks with both of my boys. The point is that even when there are two parents in the home, one parent may not feel up to the task of talking about puberty and sex. Sometimes it's better to let the more comfortable parent take the lead here, no matter the gender. But at least one parent or caregiver has to step up and lean into these topics. And I promise that whoever that is will find that once they get started, it's a lot easier than feared. The anticipation is usually worse (this applies to many things in life, and it's called anticipatory anxiety)!

Getting Mentally Prepared for These Talks

REFLECT

Before you talk to your child, I'd like you to reflect on your own journey through puberty. You may find that thinking about your child entering puberty brings back some uncomfortable memories. What went well? What didn't go well? Are there topics that are going to be triggering for you? When you reflect on your own experiences before talking to your child it gives you time to process any discomfort ahead of time.

SET AN INTENTION

Now that you've revisited your experiences and emotions as a kid going through puberty, I want you to set an intention for how you want these talks to go. Do you want to talk very openly with your partner or the child's siblings present? Do you want to have private one-on-one conversations? Do you want to use a book or bring up topics yourself? Do you want to teach your child about what is happening to the other sex? How do you want her to feel about these conversations?

For example, here's my intention with my ten- and thirteen-year-old boys. I want to speak organically about the changes in puberty, seizing opportunities when they come up, whether it's driving in the car or at home. I want to watch coming-of-age movies with them so we can talk about what the characters are going through. I want them to see things not only from their own perspective, but from other people's point of view too. I want to talk about themes related to growing up in the books they are reading. I want them to understand that puberty is not just about the physical changes, but also about social and emotional changes—and that those kinds of changes are just as important and worthy of discussion. I want them to be armed with accurate information and comfortable with coming to me with more questions. I want them to understand the why behind certain nagging things I say daily: wash your body with soap, use shampoo in your hair, brush your teeth, floss, put on deodorant, make sure you have clean underwear on, and please wear socks with shoes! I also want them to understand the why behind their changing moods and relationships, and I never want to minimize their experiences by saying, "Well, just play with someone else!" I will teach them to take deep breaths, offer a proper apology, and have hard conversations. I want to model for them taking breaks when upset and asking for a do-over. And on the days when they pass on doing something with me or they sigh when I ask yet another question or they prefer to be with their friends, I will tell them I love them, give them some space, try again later, and remind myself this is normal.

Top 10 Tips for Having "The Talk"

1. When you talk to your child, make sure to use real body part names—vagina, breasts, uterus, ovaries, menstruation, penis, testicles, sperm, semen. After you have established real names for body parts, you may also want to link them to the slang names they have so they understand they are the same body part.
2. Be ready to answer any questions your child may have. The younger you start these talks, the more questions she will likely have. The older she gets, the more embarrassed she will be. Reassure your child that no question is off-limits and that even if she feels embarrassed or shy, you promise to answer questions honestly and as best you can.
3. Keep the conversation going. There isn't just "one" talk. This should be an ongoing conversation about growth, development, changes, and the celebration of coming of age.
4. While there isn't one certain age you should start this talk, a general rule of thumb would be to start at eight for girls and nine for boys.
5. If you don't know the answer to a question, or you aren't sure what to say, just tell your kid, "That's a great question. I'm going to look into finding out the answer." Parents tend to overtalk when nervous, so just remind yourself that you can say, "I'll get back to you on that . . ." This gives you an opportunity to discuss sources of information, that some are better than others, and you can tell your child you will use information provided by doctors, hospitals, and other experts in the field.

6. Location, location, location. Where you choose to have this talk will make a big difference. You should think about where to open up this conversation (car, bedroom, on a walk) and what time (at bedtime, on a weekend morning, after school). The first talk may be preplanned or it might just happen when you find an opportune time. I like natural moments, but my experience is that parents are uncomfortable themselves so they don't always think of it or find the right moment, so initially it may be best to plan it. After that, you may want to have more casual conversations prompted by a commercial, a movie, or show to keep the conversation going.
7. If it makes you feel better, these initial talks are not about sex. They are about the changes that will occur or changes you have noticed are already occurring to her brain and body that are associated with sexual development.
8. Even if your kid has had sex ed at school, you will need to have ongoing talks. When you know it's time for health class at school, ask for a copy of the materials the kids are being taught and review it with your child at home.
9. Normalize and celebrate! Make sure you tell your child that puberty has different time frames for different kids, and that it takes years to complete. Whenever these changes start, remember it's a moment to celebrate because it means her body is doing what it should be doing.
10. Use books to help you impart this knowledge. It's good for kids to be able to look at information and formulate questions in private and from a reliable source. Some good books for girls to start with are The Care and Keeping of You series from American Girl Wellbeing. For boys, I recommend *Guy Stuff: The Body Book for Boys*, from the same publisher.

The Puberty Talk for Kids

Here are a couple of scripts to follow when you are in the right place, time, and frame of mind.

FOR GIRLS

Parent: I saw this book and thought you might want to look through it. We can read it together, or I can just leave it in your room. It talks about all the changes that happen to girls' bodies in puberty, changes you can see and changes you can't.

Child: Puberty? What's that?

Parent: Puberty is a time when your brain and body, and the brains and bodies of kids your age, change—a lot. And sometimes you might have questions about what's happening. I want you to know that I have been through this, and I want to make sure that you are ready for these changes.

Child: What do you mean? What changes?

Parent: Well, some kids are going to start growing taller. Some are going to start to develop breasts. You and your friends might have mood swings. A lot of kids will eventually get what's called acne on their faces. And when this starts to happen, your mood, your feelings, and your thoughts might change, too.

Child: Oh, okay, I think this is happening to a girl in my class, she's really tall.

Parent: Yes, that might be. Usually, the changes start in girls first, then boys go through changes, too. Puberty can even alter friendships, what you like to wear, what you want to play with, how you feel about yourself. So, knowing what's going on, and knowing that it is normal and that there's nothing wrong about this, is important.

FOR BOYS

Parent: Hey bud, I saw this book and thought you might want to look through it. We can read it together or I can just leave it in your room. It talks about all the changes that happen to boys' bodies in puberty.

Child: (uncomfortable laugh) Why would I need that?

Parent: Because around your age, boys' bodies and brains start to grow and change; some of these changes you can't see and some you can. You might have noticed that some of the girls in your class are getting taller. And some of the boys will also start growing taller, or start getting smelly feet, or even growing extra hair on their face, underarms, or legs. Have you noticed that?

Child: I don't know. I guess.

Parent: Yeah, so I just want you to know that is normal, it will happen to everyone, and sometimes you will like some of the changes, like getting bigger muscles or being stronger and faster. And sometimes you may not like some of the changes, like your voice changing or your hair getting darker, wavier, or thicker. You might even have big feelings that you don't understand.

Child: Why does that happen, and can I stop it?

Parent: This happens because there are chemicals in your body called hormones. Hormones change around this age to help you go from a boy to a teen and eventually a young man. We can't and wouldn't want to change this process because it is what the body is meant to do. It's really cool and exciting and it takes a long time to happen, so you have a couple of years to get used to these changes.

The Importance of Understanding the Connection Between Earlier Puberty and Race

In a study released in 2010, researchers found that the number of children of color going into earlier puberty was significantly higher than the number of White children. Although only 10.4 percent of White girls had developed breast buds at seven years old, over 23 percent of Black girls and almost 15 percent of Hispanic girls had developed breast buds by age seven. At eight years, 42.9 percent of Black girls, and 30.9 percent of Hispanic girls, had gotten breast buds, far higher percentages than their white peers.

Researchers believe there are a number of reasons for this disparity. Multiple studies, including results from MRI brain scans, indicate that poverty, obesity, toxic stress, and trauma are linked to physiological changes in the brain and body that can contribute, among other things, to earlier puberty. And as Black and Brown communities are disproportionately under-resourced, it follows that children growing up in those communities are more likely to be exposed to these environmental stressors that can lead them to develop early. To give just one example, in a study of childhood socioeconomic status and menstruation from 2021, socioeconomic status was a major predictor of earlier menstruation in girls.

Here's why parents, educators, and allies alike need to be concerned: children, especially girls, who develop earlier are more likely to have mental health problems, perhaps because they feel self-conscious and may be treated differently from other kids their age. In other words, earlier puberty can actually exacerbate the stress and unequal treatment of children of color.

Because of earlier puberty, too often, it's the case that Black and Brown children in particular are "adultified" in our culture. To adultify a child means to treat or consider a child as an adult, usually in a way that is wrong or harmful. In a set of four studies released in 2014, researchers found that Black boys are seen as older, more suspicious, and less innocent than their White same-age peers (the age where views of the innocence of children seemed to diverge was around age ten). In a study titled "Girlhood Interrupted: The Erasure of Black Girls' Childhood," researchers from Georgetown University shared data "showing that adults view Black girls as less innocent and more adult-like than their White peers, especially in the age range of 5–14." The consequences of this adultification can be extremely detrimental for children: the same study showed that teachers seem to spend more focus on monitoring Black girls' behavior than on encouraging their academic achievement.

We all need to understand and support children of color who may experience high levels of stress due to environmental factors and the adultification that can come from developing earlier than their peers. The first step is to protect children who look older from the unreasonable expectations of other adults, and for all of us who work with kids and around kids to watch ourselves for biases that see Black and Brown kids who go through earlier puberty as older than they are.

A TIP FOR EVERYONE: Stop viewing children who have developed early as older than they really are!

With more and more children approaching puberty at younger and younger ages, it's vitally important for everyone to be mindful of viewing kids as older than they really are. A nine-year-old child may look like she resembles a young adult, but that child is still emotionally immature—and treating her as older than she is can deprive her of her chance to develop as a child. It might feel only natural to say to a very tall ten-year-old, "Wow, you're only ten? You're a giant!" but when you comment on how grown-up she looks or make assumptions about her based on her physical maturity, you're adultifying her in ways that simply aren't fair. Let's all make a conscious choice not to do that. Resist the temptation to ask a tall kid (especially a tall Black boy) if he plays basketball. Don't ask a developing eleven-year-old girl who she has a crush on. Comments to girls like "Your parents better watch out; the boys are going to be all over you" or to boys like "I can tell you're going to break a lot of girls' hearts" sexualizes young children, adultifies them, and assumes traditional gender roles and sexual identity—it's harmful and unnecessary.

When you do want to question or comment, it's much better to focus on a child's interests, activities, and talents than her looks. If a child tells you she is ten and in fourth grade, instead of saying, "I never would have guessed! You look like a teenager already!" you can respond with "Oh, great. What's something you like about fourth grade?" As parents, our own children are watching us all the time, and when we treat other kids with this level of thoughtful respect, they will begin to follow our lead and do the same.

The Sex Script for Kids

After you have started talking to your kid about the changes that happen in puberty, naturally, you will talk to them about sexual development and reproduction. In my experience, families are in one of two camps. The first camp is the I-already-talked-to-them-about-this-in-kindergarten people who answered the "Where do babies come from?" question in a straightforward rather than baby-stork way. If this is you, great . . . and you still have work to do! They were young when you told them about eggs and sperm and fertilization, and even if they understood it, they had no personal context for it. When you have this talk again, it will make a lot more sense to them.

Perhaps you are in the we-don't-want-to-ever-talk-about-sex-with-our-kids camp. I have worked with parents who haven't discussed sex with their kids ever, and their kids are about to leave for college. I understand the feeling of awkwardness, but remember: if you don't teach them, someone else will.

So, when you have an opportune time, and you are ready, and maybe you even have some context for discussing puberty's role in sexual reproduction, here is a way you can start.

FOR GIRLS

Parent: I want to talk some more about the changes that are happening to you and your body.

Child: Okay, why?

Parent: Because while we talked about why your body was changing and how we could see some of those changes and not see others, I want to talk today about what is possible because of these changes.

Child: What do you mean? Do we really have to talk about this?

Parent: Yes, just give me a couple of minutes, I promise we don't have to talk about this all night. But I want you to understand that your body is getting ready to eventually be able to have a baby should you choose that for yourself one day.

You already know that women have eggs inside their bodies in a place called ovaries. And men have sperm in their bodies in a place called testicles. And for a baby to be made, an egg and a sperm need to meet, which happens during sex, after a man's penis goes inside a woman's vagina and he ejaculates.

What you may not know is that a boy's body doesn't make sperm until he goes through puberty. And before a girl goes through puberty, her eggs are just waiting. Then, toward the end of puberty, her ovaries start releasing one egg every month to go down the fallopian tubes to the uterus. The uterus builds up a lining to welcome that egg so it can grow into a baby. If an egg isn't fertilized, the blood flows out of the vagina. That is called a menstrual cycle.

I know it might sound scary, but I will teach you how to use a pad and stay clean before it happens. And getting your period is a good thing, because it means that someday, when you are a grown-up and if you want to, you can have a baby.

Your daughter's reaction will vary greatly from tears, to avoidance, to more questions—so at this point be ready for anything.

FOR BOYS

Parent: I want to talk to you more about the changes that are happening to you and your body.

Child: Okay, why?

Parent: Because while we talked about why your body was changing and how we could see some of those changes and not see others, I want to talk today about what is possible because of these changes.

Child: What do you mean? Do we really have to talk about this?

Parent: Yes, just give me a couple of minutes, I promise we don't have to talk about this all night, but I want you to understand that your body is getting ready so that when you are a man, you can have a baby with a woman, if you both want to.

You already know that women have eggs inside their bodies in a place called ovaries. And men have sperm in their bodies in a place called testicles. And for a baby to be made, egg and sperm need to meet, which happens during sex when a man's penis goes inside a woman's vagina.

What you may not know is that a boy's body doesn't make sperm until puberty. And a girl's body doesn't release any eggs until puberty. So puberty is what makes it possible for a man and a woman to make a baby when they have sex.

Remember, this is the first of many conversations, so if you feel like you have stumbled or missed a point—don't panic! You will have plenty of opportunities to talk about it again.

What If Your Child Comes to You with Questions?

If your child approaches you with concern about a bodily change, start by clarifying what she is asking you (this is a good strategy in any communication). Repeat in your own words what you hear her asking you, until she says that is in fact what she *was* asking. Once you know that, you can begin a dialogue:

> **Parent:** Okay, so what I'm hearing is that you want to know why no one else is as tall as you are in the third grade. That's a good question with a couple of possible answers. First, it could be something that all kids go through, which is a time called puberty. During this time, your brain says to your body that it's time to start growing into an adult, and your body says, "Okay!" and starts changing. This can start anytime for you or any one of your friends from now until about the end of middle school. For you, it seems it may be starting now.
>
> **Child:** What does that mean?
>
> **Parent:** It means you may grow and become taller than other kids your age for a while. It means you might change your mind about the things you like to do or play with. It's all okay; it will happen to everyone over the next few years, and at the end of that time, you will all wind up the height, size, and person who you are meant to be. (Add the following, if true.) Plus, you should know that I went through puberty when I was about your age too. I remember feeling (add whatever you truly felt).

Child: But the kids in class sometimes say mean things to me, like I look like a giraffe.

Parent: I'm really sorry to hear this. Sometimes kids can say mean things when they don't understand something. Maybe if they understood that it's normal for kids to grow and change at different ages and grades that would help everyone accept and be nice to each other more.

Child: Yeah, maybe. What should I do?

Parent: Well, first I want you to start with you. I want you to celebrate this time and learn about it because the more comfortable you are with yourself, and your changing brain and body, the easier it will be for you when you are around other kids who may not understand.

Rather than sitting your child down and overwhelming him with too much information, I suggest you talk to him a little bit at a time about body changes in the order he will likely experience them. I don't think it's too early to talk to an eight-year-old boy about the earliest sign of puberty, which is an enlarged scrotum, and for girls, breast buds. Each talk should offer information about what's happening, and perhaps end with a hint about what's next. So, for example, you might say, "This is just the beginning of growing up, and a few months after this starts, you might hit a growth spurt. We can talk more about that another time."

HEIGHT AND WEIGHT

One unmistakable sign of puberty for both sexes is a growth spurt. After the steady growth of middle childhood, girls start shooting up around age nine, while boys start rapid growth around age eleven. Over two and a half years, girls grow an average of eleven inches; boys grow about twelve inches over three years.[2]

Rapidly growing children often experience benign pains in their limbs that their parents might have known as "growing pains." Interestingly, research hasn't pinned down exactly what the pains are or why they occur—or even whether growth is a factor at all. But if the pain is sporadic and doesn't keep a child from his usual activities, it probably falls into that "growing pains" category.

Weight changes as well. During puberty the average child gains about 6.5 pounds a year, and body fat increases. In girls, the weight tends to go to their breasts and hips, and their new curves can make them self-conscious. Boys generally don't mind the weight gain as much; looking bigger helps them feel stronger and more confident.

Your child may ask if his height and weight are normal for his age. You might be able to answer this question by pointing out your own growth patterns at that age and explaining that often height and weight can be genetic. Or you can say that this is something you can talk to the pediatrician about next time you're due for a visit.

BODY ODOR

Kids in middle childhood don't seem to notice or care about body odor! I learned this the hard way, when I first started seeing tweens and teens in a space in my office called the swing room, which is outfitted with hanging fabric that kids can climb and swing on, or curl up in. I would ask the child I was meeting with to take off shoes to play on the swings and would gag at the smell from the shoes, socks, and feet (it's not a very large space)! I now make light of the stench, to normalize it, and then use it as a teachable moment to discuss puberty and body odor: Did you know humans have more sweat glands on the soles of the feet than anywhere else?

Curiously, while kids this age don't seem to be sensitive about their foot or armpit odor, they're often into body sprays, which they seem to assume make them attractive. Many tween girls love places like Bath & Body Works; when they become teens, they graduate to actual perfume sold by celebrities and influencers, often costing vast amounts of money.[3] Boys are also affected by the body spray trend; at ten, my younger son asked to get Axe, which has been around for forty years.[4]

With puberty arriving earlier, kids are getting stinky earlier, and many parents tell me about how surprised they are to get a whiff of their eight-year-old that brings them right back to their middle school PE locker room days. Even if you think your child is too young for smelliness caused by puberty, it's best to address it with your child, rather than ignoring it. You really don't want someone else announcing to your kid that he smells, which could wind up shaming him. By presenting this as a normal part of growing up—and providing kids with deodorant and basic hygiene reminders—your child will see this change as unremarkable and something that's easy to deal with.

Girls in my puberty classes will sometimes say to me, "My parents don't want me to use antiperspirant yet." Some parents are concerned about studies that have linked antiperspirant use to breast cancer. According to the Cleveland Clinic, no extensive studies have researched the potential connection between breast cancer and deodorants. Many smaller, limited studies have, however, and the results of these studies have not shown any clear relationship between the use of deodorants and antiperspirants and breast cancer. Still, when a parent and child ask what they can do because of their concerns, I tell these parents that aluminum-free products are available, as well as natural and organic lines that say they don't contain harmful chemicals.

Here is a sample script for talking to kids about body odor:

Parent: I want to talk to you about the new smells that are coming from your body. Have you noticed that this is happening to you sometimes?

Child: No, what do you mean?

Parent: Well, now that you are getting older and are starting puberty, you're beginning to sweat more than you used to in sports or on hot days, and you also may sweat when you are embarrassed or are having big feelings, just like I do.

Child: Oh, okay.

Parent: So, there might be times when the sweat under your armpits or on your feet might smell bad. When that happens, I might ask you to take a shower. I'm doing this so that you get clean and so that we are all comfortable in the house. Taking showers every day with soap and shampoo will help with this.

Child: I *do* take baths or showers.

Parent: That's true, and it will be more important than ever that you really clean your skin and head with soap and shampoo when you are showering, and maybe use a washcloth. Then, when you get out you should put on clean clothes and deodorant or antiperspirant and wash the stinky clothes. This will help control your sweating and the smell. I do this, too.

After a talk like this, the next time you're with your kid at a store you can explain the difference between antiperspirants (which protects against sweat and odor) and deodorants (which cover up odor) and have them pick out a product they want to try with your approval.

HAIR

Hair is a major focus of kids in puberty, first as it starts to grow and then as they start to consider getting rid of it. During puberty, girls and boys get pubic hair and underarm hair and their leg hair becomes thicker and darker.

You should know that many of the girls in my classes seem to think that pubic hair is supposed to be eliminated, and they're very much aware of procedures such as Brazilian waxes. I tell them that, just like our eyebrows, eyelashes, and nostril hairs, pubic hair serves a protective function. It traps dirt, debris, and bacteria that can cause infections. It can also reduce friction during athletic activities. I add that the skin in that area is very sensitive and advise them that if they decide to wax when they are older, they should go to a professional.

Girls can also get some darker hair above their lips, and their eyebrows may continue to grow thicker and wider. Some girls may want to wax or bleach or pluck this facial hair, and, if so, I suggest that parents take them to a professional when/if they are comfortable, as well.

Boys will start to grow facial hair at some point in late puberty. At first it may grow patchily above the upper lip, then it will get thicker, darker, and spread evenly above the lip. Eventually, it will spread to the cheeks, chin, and neck, but again, this may occur erratically.

It's not unheard of for an eleven- or twelve-year-old boy to want to shave. You or another trusted adult should guide your son through this sort of rite of passage, offering up information about shaving cream, razors (including proper cleaning and storage), and post-shave skin care. Issues like razor burn, cuts, and ingrown hairs can really cause irritation and discomfort for boys in puberty.

Girls don't usually start to grow armpit hair until closer to the end of puberty, but they may get curious about shaving their legs earlier on. The age at which a girl may want to start shaving can vary greatly. I don't think there's a right or wrong answer about whether a girl shaves; it's really about her personal preference and readiness. I encourage you to discuss the pros and cons with your daughter, as I do in my classes; you may find that it leads to other relevant topics of conversation. If your daughter does decide to shave, in addition to teaching her how to do it safely, emphasize that she should not share razors because of the risk of infection.

Boys don't have as many issues with hair at this age. Toward the end of middle childhood, they might ask for hair products. And when they are teens, they are often on the eager lookout for chest hair, which may not develop until they are in their late teens or even their twenties.

Both boys and girls can suffer from oily hair starting in puberty, however, which can also cause self-consciousness. Each hair follicle has its own oil gland, and during puberty these glands produce more oil. Washing hair daily or with a shampoo formulated for oily hair can help.

BOYS' REPRODUCTIVE SYSTEM

Along with those first sparse pubertal hairs for boys, one of the earliest signs of puberty is changes in the size of their genitals. This growth is mostly due to increased production of testosterone. It also often happens out of parents' sight, because, naturally, as boys grow older, they no longer walk around naked or need help bathing.

These changes start around age ten, so I advise parents to discuss them before that. Again, use the proper terms. You can tell your son his genital area is made up of his penis and scrotum, and that the latter contains two testicles, where sperm are made. Both his penis and his scrotum are going to grow in the next few years, and it may be something that he may or may not notice because it is usually gradual.

Boys in puberty may ask questions about the size of their penis. Educate your son that the rate of penis growth and final size is genetic. Reassure him that penis size is just a difference like hair color, one is not better than the other—they're just different.

Another difference in penises that your son may or may not become aware of is whether they are circumcised. You can explain that circumcision is the surgical removal of a newborn boy's foreskin, which is the skin on the tip of the penis. The procedure is common for newborn boys in certain parts of the world, including the United States. For some families, circumcision is a religious ritual. The procedure can also be a matter of family tradition, personal hygiene, or preventive health care. Emphasize that it's a personal choice.

At some point, you may notice that your son wants privacy, or asks for extra time to get out of bed in the morning. This could be because he is experiencing erections, another result of increased testosterone production. Boys can experience erections at any age, but they happen more often in puberty.

Boys used to hearing the term "boner" are often surprised to learn that there are no bones in the penis, and that it is made up of tissue and blood vessels. I encourage parents to demystify erections by explaining that they occur when increased blood flow fills up the tissue in the penis, changing its shape from mainly soft and bent to hard and upright (it might help to explain that erect means rigidly upright). Erections can occur when a person is sleeping, shortly before they awaken, when they are thinking about certain things, or for what seems like no reason at all. Assure your son that unpredictable erections are normal and that this stage won't last forever. In addition, the more erections he gets, the more comfortable he will become with them and the more he will learn how to handle them, and perhaps even predict what triggers them.

Ejaculation can be a particularly uncomfortable topic for parents to talk about with their sons, but if you keep it scientific, it doesn't have to be too embarrassing for you or your child. In fact, it's just a continuation of earlier conversations about sexual reproduction, when you discussed sperm but probably not semen. So remind your son that a sperm cell fertilizes an egg cell to produce a baby. Then explain that the way sperm cells get out of the penis is via a fluid called semen, which can appear clear or cloudy. And the term for when semen comes out of the penis is "ejaculation." This can lead to a discussion of ejaculations as purposeful or involuntary. When I think a boy is ready, or when they ask, I explain to them that the slang term "jerking off" means to tug on their own penis because it feels good—so good that it can result in ejaculation. I also explain that the formal term for this is "masturbation" (almost 100 percent of boys by age fifteen will have masturbated to ejaculation).[5]

An involuntary ejaculation, I tell them, occurs when semen comes out of their penis at night while they are sleeping. They may have heard this called a "wet dream"; I also explain that the formal term is "nocturnal emission." (Sometimes it's helpful for kids to know that bodily functions that they consider embarrassing are so commonplace as to have very boring scientific-sounding names.) Boys find it reassuring to know that this is normal. If a boy hasn't been educated and is afraid to ask, he may think it's urine, which is why I advise having this talk before it occurs.

Fun Fact: Shortly after I started writing this book my fifth-grade son had two days of sexual education at his school. When he came home on the first day, I asked him what he learned that was new to him. With ease, he said, "I didn't know that you can wake up with wet stuff in your underwear." He kind of smiled and said that was about it. I noted to myself that I'd be sure to include this story in my book so you'd know that even though I teach this and talk about it openly, I hadn't covered everything by fifth grade, and that's fine!

Another way to normalize this experience is to tell him what to do when ejaculation occurs: simply put their sheets or pajamas in the wash (I recommend having a few sets of each) and find fresh ones. Don't ask or question him about why there's no sheet on the bed or excess laundry. Granting him privacy and respecting his changing body is an essential tool in your parenting kit.

MASTURBATION

It may be helpful for you to recall that fondling of one's own private parts starts sometimes with a baby or toddler who discovers their penis.

From birth to age two, both boys and girls explore their bodies, including the genital areas. Infant and toddler boys can experience erections, and girls can produce vaginal lubricant. By preschool ages (three to four) they become aware of and curious about gender and body differences. This is when they may begin to play doctor or mommy and daddy with friends or siblings. From kindergarten through second grade (about ages five to seven), children can continue to play out sexual gender roles, and they may get curious about pregnancy and birthing.

Ages eight to twelve usher in puberty at different rates. During this time, children will start to develop a sense of privacy—and their first crushes. As uncomfortable as it may be for parents to accept, children in this age range of middle childhood may masturbate to ejaculation. Toward middle school, ages eleven or twelve, kids may fantasize about celebrities, adults, or other teens in a sexualized way. Again, it is all a normal part of child development.

VOICE CHANGES AND ADAM'S APPLES

The larynx (voice box) grows in both boys and girls during puberty, and the vocal folds (formerly known as cords) lengthen and thicken. But this happens to a greater degree, and more noticeably, for boys, whose voices deepen about an octave compared with a third of an octave for girls.[6] While boy's vocal folds—which are muscles—adapt to these changes, their voices sometimes warble and crack. This stage typically lasts weeks to months and then the voice settles in at its new pitch.

In boys, the larynx grows so much that the protective cartilage in front of it forms what looks like a lump in the throat. This is known colloquially as an Adam's apple.

GIRLS' BREAST DEVELOPMENT

One of the very first signs of puberty in girls is breast buds. They are small bumps that appear right under the nipple and can feel tender. If a child is not prepared for breast buds to show up—and does not understand that they can appear in one breast and not the other and grow unevenly—the experience can be concerning or isolating for them. Because breast buds are now appearing in girls as young as eight years old, it's important that you talk about it before then.

Even if girls know what to expect they still might not welcome breast development, or be especially sensitive if they're the first to develop or if they feel unsure about their gender identity. Girls in the early stages may often start wearing loose tops or tugging at their shirts. Some have even asked me if there is anything they can do to stop breast development. Breast growth can be slow, uncomfortable, and awkward, and breast buds (about the size of a blueberry) have been known to come and go before actually fully developing.

When you explain these stages to your daughter, use the proper words and definitions and be matter-of-fact about the reproductive purpose of breasts—to nurse a baby, should she ever want to. A nipple is the part of the breast where milk can be released. Like breasts, nipples can come in different shapes. They also come in a range of colors, from pale pink to dark brown. The areola is the circular area of dark and bumpy skin around the nipple (the bumps are lubricating glands). The milk glands produce milk, and the milk ducts carry the milk to the nipple.

This swelling and growth are signs that breasts are developing milk glands. Fat and connective tissue grow around the milk glands to protect them, which give breasts their adult shape and size. Breasts can be big or small, round or pointy, high or low, pointing up or down, even or uneven. There is no perfect breast shape or size.

And your daughter's breasts may not look like yours. While genetics play a significant role in breast development (remember, those genes can come from the father's side, too!), other factors include hormones, weight, nutrition, and environmental toxins.

As you and your daughter might have read in the book *Are You There God? It's Me, Margaret*, or seen in the movie, girls used to do all kinds of exercises to try to make their breasts larger. It might be a good idea to tell your daughter, "That book was written a really long time ago, when people thought that things like exercise could make their breasts grow." It gave girls a sense of control over what seems like an uncontrollable process. When I was that age I believed it, too! But we now know that the way your breasts develop is mostly due to genetics.

This is also a good time to assure your daughter that whatever her breasts end up looking like, their size will have nothing to do with how well she can nurse a baby, how feminine she is, how attractive people will find her, or what sports she can play. Also let her know that even when she's grown, they will still change shape and size.

Girls sometimes ask me to help them tell their parents they want a bra, and parents' reactions run the gamut from "Do you really think you need a bra?" to "I already have one for you." (If you are wondering why your flat-chested child wants a bra, I have treated girls who just want to stuff them or to feel older.)

If you aren't sure your daughter needs a bra, you can ask these questions:

- Are your breasts showing through shirts?
- Do you feel pain or self-consciousness when you play sports because of soreness or bouncing or chafing?
- Would you be more comfortable with an extra layer?

BOYS AND BREASTS (YES!)

Up to 70 percent of boys in early to mid-puberty experience gynecomastia, which is enlarged male breast tissue caused by normal hormonal changes in puberty. This can start as early as age ten, with a peak onset between the ages of thirteen and fourteen. By age seventeen, when hormones tend to level out, only about 10 percent of boys still have enlarged breast tissue.

You might not observe this directly. A couple of telltale signs are boys who wear oversize shirts or who don't want to go swimming. Be reassuring and supportive. Let your son know that this is a temporary situation and ask if there's anything that would make him more comfortable in the pool or ocean (wearing a swim shirt or rash guard, perhaps). Never force him to join you. Simply say something like "I understand how you feel. We're all going to go into the water, and I'd love to see you if you change your mind." Then don't make a big deal about it if he does join you.

GIRLS' REPRODUCTIVE SYSTEM

Far too often, girls are told that the name for their genitals is simply the vagina. I tell girls in my classes the proper names for their reproductive body parts. I also divide the body parts into the internal reproductive organs—the parts of the body that make it possible for a person to have a baby (reproduce) and the outer parts, the genitals, which I also refer to as their private parts. Boys and girls should be educated on both reproductive systems.

Internal Reproductive Parts: The Basics

Ovaries: These are two roundish organs on either side of a girl's pelvis that contain egg cells. On the day a baby girl is born, she has over one million eggs, about the size of the tip of a needle in her ovaries. When she turns ten, she will have about 300,000 eggs left—the eggs have been dying off on daily basis since she was born.

Fallopian tubes: These tiny tubes, about four inches long and as thin as a strand of spaghetti, guide the egg to the uterus.

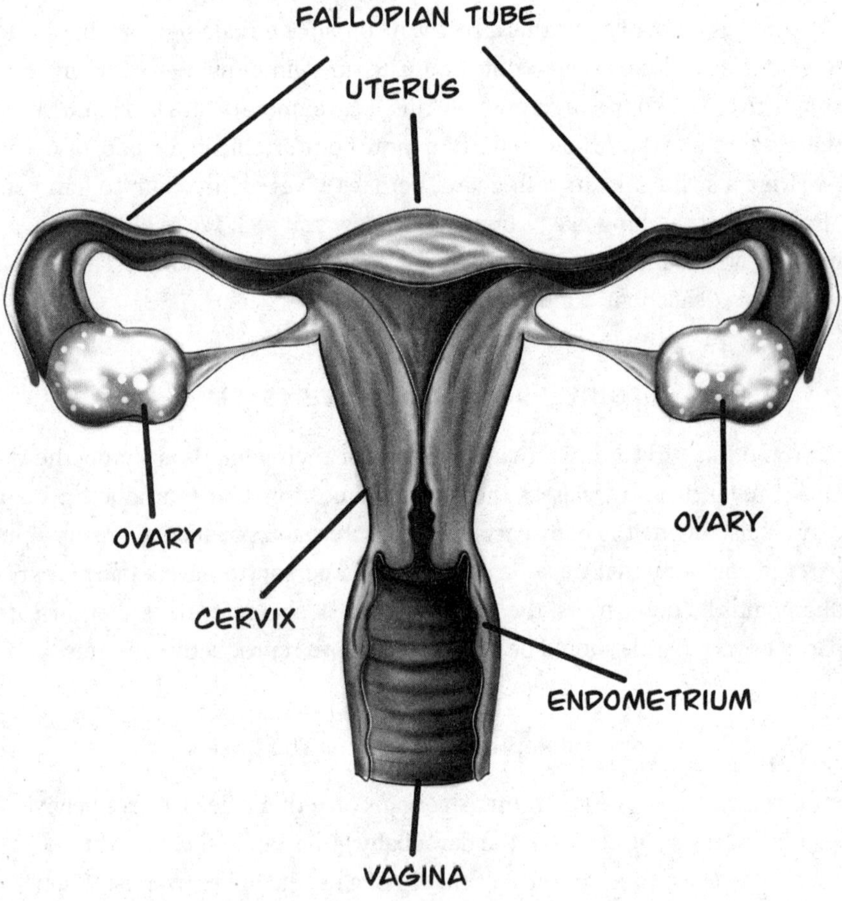
FALLOPIAN TUBE
UTERUS
OVARY
OVARY
CERVIX
ENDOMETRIUM
VAGINA

Uterus: Also called the womb, this organ is an upside-down triangle between your fallopian tubes and it is where a fertilized egg develops into a baby. It's about the size of a fist in a woman and stretches with the growing baby.

Cervix: The bottom of the uterus. Its purpose is to protect the inside of the uterus and to provide an opening between the uterus and the vagina.

Vagina: This is the passageway into and out of a woman's reproductive organs. Sperm travel up the vagina, through the cervix and uterus, and into the fallopian tubes. If there is an egg in the fallopian tube, it could become fertilized by sperm and move to the uterus to grow into a baby. When a baby is in the process of being born, it travels from the uterus through the cervix and out the vagina.

External Reproductive Parts

The outer and inner lips (also known as labia) protect the delicate reproductive parts inside. The vaginal opening is the entrance to the vagina, and the urethra opening is where pee comes out of your body. The clitoris is a small, sensitive spot that can make you feel good when touched.

Girls' genitals do not change as much as boys' during puberty. The vulva grows along with the rest of her body and becomes more pigmented. But about a year after breast buds appear, girls may notice a clear or whitish fluid in their underwear. This fluid is called vaginal discharge, and most often starts appearing six months to one year before menstruation begins. The amount that girls report noticing this can vary greatly.

Vaginal discharge has the important role of keeping the vagina clean. Discharge is made up of fluid to keep the vagina moist, and healthy bacteria to fight off bad bacteria. It does not usually stain underwear if washed, or typically smell, but some girls are uncomfortable with the moisture and may wear a liner. Once menstruation begins, discharge will continue to be a part of being a young woman throughout adulthood. The consistency of the discharge, however, will change throughout each cycle based on hormonal changes occurring in the body. Generally, nothing needs to be done for discharge unless pain, itching, or a foul odor is noted, in which case an appointment to the pediatrician is advised.

ACNE

Acne during puberty is a common skin condition where the skin becomes blemished. It is primarily due to the hormonal changes associated with puberty, particularly an increase in androgens, which are male sex hormones (though they are present in both boys and girls). Testosterone is an androgen, and when it rises, it stimulates the sebaceous (oil) glands in the skin to produce more sebum, an oily substance. This excess sebum can mix with dead skin cells and clog hair follicles, leading to the development of acne, which can show up as blackheads, whiteheads, cysts, or pimples.

Approximately 85 to 90 percent of teenagers have this common skin problem, but only about 20 percent of kids in middle childhood develop acne. However, I've known girls as young as third grade who had visible bumps.

If you or your child's father had acne, it's very likely that your child will too, and this will give you a good idea about if you need to prepare for this. Good hygiene and a new skin care routine become important factors in managing acne during puberty. I recommend a matter-of-fact, here's-what-we-are-going-to-do-about-it approach, while not downplaying your child's concerns.

I find it important to talk to the kids in my practice about what to do because they often get bad advice from friends and TikTok. I've had kids tell me they were using rubbing alcohol to clean their faces or toothpaste on their pimples. While neither of these ideas are necessarily harmful, there are much more gentle and effective products.

Here's a script for talking about acne with your child:

Parent: You know how we've talked about how at this stage in your life your hormones are changing and causing changes in you, some of which you might like and some of which you might not like?

Child: Yeah, why?

Parent: I've noticed that you have some acne on your face. That's because oil glands get stimulated when hormones are active. Also, acne is genetic, and I had it when I was in puberty too.

At this point, you should be prepared for a range of responses and emotions. Stay calm in the moment. You might hear any of the following, even if your child is upset about the acne and does want help:

Child: I don't care.

or

Oh my God, Mom! Why do you care? Why do you have to bring this stuff up? You think hormones cause everything and you are *so annoying and embarrassing*. Leave me alone!

or

I hate my face.

or

What should I do?

Parent: (calmly) We don't have to talk more about this now, but if it ever bothers you, I am happy to share products and hygiene routines that can be helpful.

or

Now is a good time to start a good skin care routine. I know this is new, but once you do it a few times it will become easier. I can get you some products, or you can come with me. Just let me know.

If your child says they "hate their face," a helpful response to that is, in a calm voice, to let them know that you hear him. You don't want to minimize his feelings by saying something like "but you're so handsome!" (You can say that at other times.) Instead, say, "I hear you: You're really upset about the way your face is being affected by these changes in puberty. I know it probably feels scary and like you don't know what to do. I promise you this is a stage. It won't last forever, and your face will be clear again."

MENSTRUATION

How parents handle the subject of menstruation has a lasting impact on their daughters, like Andie, an eleven-year-old girl whose parents were divorced. No one had ever talked to Andie about her period, so when hers started she coped the best she could, hiding her bloody underwear and wads of toilet paper in the trash. After about three months of this, Andie's stepmother found some stained tissue in a wastebasket. Andie insisted she had a bloody nose before reluctantly acknowledging that she had gotten her period and didn't feel comfortable going to her mother, father, or stepmother. Why had no one talked to this child? Her mother thought Andie had learned about periods in school and assumed she would come to her for guidance. Her stepmother hadn't felt it was her place to speak to Andie. Her father, who never had sisters and had no other daughters, said he didn't think it was an issue he should—or could—take on. So, here was a kid with three parental figures whose introduction to menstruation was a story of abandonment, embarrassment, and fear. Not the way you want a kid to enter young womanhood.

Nine-year-old Gabby, on the other hand, was well prepared. Her mother had talked to her well before Gabby got her period at an especially awkward moment—during a swim meet. Gabby asked her mom if she could swim in the race (she could and did, and there was no huge trail of blood) and then as a matter of fact put on a pad afterward. From the get-go, this girl's attitude was "Just tell me what to do" and so she felt confident she could handle it. Hers was a story of empowerment. The next time I saw her, she eagerly told me, "I am a woman now!" and mused about renegotiating her bedtime.

In my classes, I encourage parents to prepare girls for periods by giving them a cute but nondescript "period pouch" (that could be a pencil case) and putting some deodorant, a pad, an extra pair of underwear, and a liner, along with a piece of candy for comfort. By carrying the pouch around in her backpack, your daughter will feel ready if she gets her first period during the school day.

Explaining menstruation to a tween can be a sensitive and important conversation. Here are some tips to help you do so in a clear and supportive way. Remember, if you're reading this and your daughter has already gotten her period, it's not too late! You can still find opportunities to have these kinds of conversations with your child.

As with the puberty/sexual reproduction talks, choose the right time and place. Use age-appropriate language. Tailor your words and message to your child's level. As noted before, you should avoid using euphemisms, use proper terms, and explain slang where necessary.

- **Start with the basics.** Begin by explaining what menstruation is in simple terms. You can say something like "Menstruation (or getting your period) is a natural part of becoming a young woman. It's the process where your body prepares for the possibility of pregnancy each month. I know this sounds kind of silly since that is so far off for you, but your amazing body wants a lot of practice."
- **Explain the menstrual cycle.** Outline the monthly release of an egg into the fallopian tube (ovulation), and the buildup up of the uterine lining to nourish the egg if it is fertilized. Explain that if the egg isn't fertilized, the body sheds the uterine lining through the vagina (menstruation). Yes, I use all those terms, and they understand. Illustrations, which you can find online or in a book, help as well.
- **Address emotions.** Make sure you discuss both the ones they might feel in the moment (I've seen it all: awkwardness, disgust, sadness, anxiety, excitement) and the moodiness that getting a period can elicit. Provide accurate information and reassurance. If this has happened earlier than you expected, remember, it's still within the norm; try to keep any shock or sorrow from your child. Girls often feel like they are the first to get their period, and that "everyone knows." You can point out that you have no idea about the other girls in their class; some girls like to share, and some don't. Tell your daughter it's her private information and she should only share it if she truly wants to, and with a trusted friend.
- **Discuss the signs.** Signals such as abdominal cramps, bloating, facial breakouts, sore breasts, and mood changes indicate a period might be coming. Mention that periods can last for a full week and can start with

spotting, then heavier flow, and go back to spotting before it stops. Blood color can range from a kind of rusty brown to light pink.
- **Talk about hygiene.** Discuss and demonstrate the use of sanitary products like pads or tampons; don't assume your child knows what "wings" are. Tell them how often tampons need to be changed to prevent toxic shock syndrome. I advise younger girls to wait for a year before they use tampons to allow their cycle to become regular and especially because I don't think nine- or ten-year-olds can keep track of changing tampons within the recommended time frame.
- **Normalize the experience.** Let your child know that menstruation is a normal part of life, and it's experienced by millions of people around the world. Share personal stories or anecdotes. Watch coming-of-age movies such as *Turning Red*. This goes for dads as well. Girls can sometimes be sensitive about their fathers knowing that they've gotten their periods. Dads don't need to make a big deal of it; a quiet acknowledgment of this milestone is fine. And they should show that they are comfortable with this fact of life. Girls should not feel awkward about telling their fathers they are out of pads, or that they have cramps and would like someone to bring them a heating pad and some Tylenol. The message from Dad should be "I know that you have gotten your period, and I'm here to support you in any way that I can."
- **Be mindful in divorced or blended households.** In the case of divorce, make sure your daughter has supplies in each home. In the case of blended households, you should know that studies have shown that girls who live with an unrelated male get their period earlier, this is referred to as the "male effect."[7] This is believed to be influenced by the regular presence of a nonbiological male, which can lead to hormonal changes in the girl. The exact reasons are not fully understood, but it is thought that their presence may accelerate the timing of puberty due to pheromonal cues, which are chemical signals that can affect hormone levels and developmental timing.
- **Offer ongoing support.** Remember this conversation is just the beginning of many. Ensure that your daughter knows she can always come to you with questions or concerns as she continues to deal with changes in her body. It's essential to maintain open communication and provide ongoing support as the tween navigates the changes in their body during adolescence.

- **Mark the occasion.** Talk about how you want to celebrate this milestone. It could be with a small piece of jewelry, a special meal, anything that acknowledges she's a growing girl.

Coping Strategies to Help You and Your Child Navigate the Changes of Earlier Puberty

While you want your child to understand and not be ashamed of starting puberty on the earlier side, it's also important to ensure that your child still gets to enjoy the fullness of their childhood. Here are some coping strategies to help you and your child navigate this time.

- Talk to your child about the changes that are occurring in categories—social, emotional, physical, and cognitive. For example, you can say, "Even though your body is growing bigger (physical), you may still want to play with things (cognitive and emotional) like you did when your body was smaller, and that's normal." It can help your child maintain age-appropriate interests and activities.
- Advocate. If you know that your child is going through earlier puberty, you will need to talk to teachers, coaches, and family members about still treating your child in a way that suits her chronological age. It's very likely this conversation will need to be repeated over time. You can say something like "Hey Coach, Tommy has recently gone through a huge growth spurt, and I notice that sometimes other people, his teachers, and even we as his parents treat him like he's older than he actually is. I just wanted to share that we are working hard at remembering that he is just eleven and appreciate any efforts you and your staff can put in at trying to do the same, too. We don't want him to feel like he has to grow up too fast just because he's physically bigger than other kids right now."
- Continue age-appropriate exposure. If your child is immersed in age-appropriate games, toys, and shows, it will keep her grounded in childhood—it's when kids are exposed to content meant for older people that they can become confused, distressed, or desensitized.

Puberty is a complicated process to begin with. The fact that it's happening earlier, overlapping with the middle childhood years, is a change that is worthy of concern. But it also offers you opportunities as a parent. By focusing on your child's mental health now, you can help her not only get through puberty in a more positive and informed way but can provide her with the habits and resilience that will get her safely through adolescence.

PART II

The Foundation of a Healthy Relationship

CHAPTER 3

The Unexpected Ups and Downs of Middle Childhood

What Parents Can Do to Help

Be kind, for everyone you meet is fighting a hard battle.

—Plato

Not so long ago, I received an email from a mother named Jaime. "We're really struggling and could use some direction," she wrote in her message, explaining that her son Ryan, who was nine years old and in third grade at the time, was struggling. "Ryan is getting upset on a daily basis before school. After school, he's hit the babysitter, he doesn't listen to us, he fights every transition. As parents, we set boundaries and our younger child is happy to follow them, but no matter how many consequences we give Ryan, he refuses to comply. We're out of ideas. Nothing is working!"

Later, when I followed up with Jaime on the phone, I learned that the family had recently moved to the area and Jaime had just given birth to a third child. Ryan had started his new school that September, and although he seemed to have gotten off to a good start, before long, he was bursting into tears at the beginning of each school day. Jaime told me she had to beg Ryan to get out of the car and into the classroom, where he stayed upset much longer than is typical for a third grader. Even when Ryan calmed down, his teachers reported that he remained sullen and unfocused; he'd reply when called on but wouldn't proactively engage in classroom activities or discussions. Meanwhile, Jaime was spending her days at work worrying about how Ryan was doing at school and if he had stopped crying yet. "It's like having a preschooler again," she observed. "Aren't we supposed to have moved past this by now? I just don't know what to do."

Ryan's dad, Greg, was concerned about Ryan as well—and worried about his wife as he thought she was being too hard on herself. What both parents agreed about was that it was increasingly difficult to predict when Ryan would be able to cope with everyday demands and when he wouldn't. If Jaime needed to run an errand on the way home, Ryan would often become irritable and upset, and before she knew it, Ryan was having a full-on meltdown. If he asked to stop for ice cream and she refused, he would start kicking and pounding the driver's seat until she gave in. Mealtimes had also become a minefield. If Ryan didn't get mac and cheese, chicken nuggets, or pizza, he'd physically flop to the ground in protest.

Jaime was exhausted. She felt like a bad mother because it seemed like all her energy was going toward Ryan while neglecting her other children. It was taking every last ounce of her energy to raise him and she was worried about his future. "When he's not this way," she told me, "he's the sweetest thing. But when he gets upset, it's really hard to get him back on track—and he stays that way for much longer than he used to do, even compared to when he was a toddler."

The fact is, between ages six and twelve, kids have a lot going on. Hormonal changes and transitions in the brain are beginning; these can cause emotions to become more intense and unpredictable, with some children lashing out or internalizing their unhappiness. Girls can become more self-conscious and insecure. Boys often become more aggressive. Shame is an intense emotion that can also come into play, especially around looks, performance, and changing bodies. Sleep patterns may shift, affecting your child's bedtime and ability to cope during the day. Expectations at school and home are amping up as well, with kids responding to new social and academic pressures with increased stress. In addition to being moody, children who are already on the sensitive side may become easily offended or embarrassed. This is a time of great vulnerability in a child's life, when he can feel as if everything is out of his control.

It's a difficult phase for parents as well. All of a sudden, your formerly sweet and snuggly child may want more independence from you. He'll start wanting to spend more time with his friends. He may also push for his privacy—preferring to be alone in his room or playing video games. You may experience feelings of loss as a result, and it may seem as if you're being robbed of time with your kid. "I didn't know this would happen this early" is a refrain I hear from so many parents.

As children enter the early middle childhood years (ages six to eight), they are generally working on their emotional regulation skills like calming themselves down, expressing emotions verbally, and frustration tolerance. It's typical for them to still struggle with expressing big feelings, especially with the increased demands of a full school day. In the later middle childhood years (ages nine to twelve) children typically show gains in emotional regulation, becoming more mature. Common issues such as friendships, increased academic pressures, increased complex and dynamic emotions, and the onset of puberty may contribute to moodiness, outbursts, or the occasional meltdown. The key word is "occasional." If your child's moodiness is more frequent, as it was with Ryan, it may mean that he needs more support from you.

As I explained to Jaime, the first thing to understand is that earlier puberty is likely playing a role. Moods in middle childhood can be *even more* labile than in the teenage years. Remember, puberty starts first in the brain, not in the body.

Jaime and Greg had tried everything with Ryan: negotiating, time-outs, counting down, five-minute warnings, all of which eventually turned into bribery, empty threats, yelling, giving in, and giving up. In fact, there was good reason why they weren't having any success. What Ryan was experiencing was something called "emotional dysregulation," which is a technical term for out-of-proportion anger, irritability, rigidity, moodiness, volatility, and unpredictable behavior.

The term "emotional dysregulation" has been around for a long time in academia, but it's only more recently begun appearing in mainstream conversations around kids and parents. The phrase was coined by Dr. Marsha Linehan, the psychologist who developed dialectical behavior therapy (DBT), while working with adults with borderline personality disorder who were struggling to manage their emotions and navigate relationships and friendships. Here's how I explain it to my clients: emotional dysregulation is when a child is unable to respond to the demands of his day in a way that's flexible, controlled, and socially acceptable. Children who are emotionally dysregulated are also often referred to as highly sensitive or difficult. They cry easily and get agitated by what most people deem to be small things.

"When a child is emotionally dysregulated," I explained to Jaime and Greg, "he needs something very different from punishment, consequences, or incentives. Ryan needs to understand his emotions and then manage them . . . and as his parent, you can help him to do that. Once he's better able to control his emotions, you'll find that it's a lot easier to set boundaries and have him follow them."

Emotional dysregulation can take many different forms. In Ryan's case, it manifested as a kind of chronic moodiness and outsize reactions to everyday situations. For other kids, it can result in outbursts that seem to appear from nowhere. You may have a kid who is easygoing 90 percent of the time, but then something happens—he doesn't get to eat all the Halloween candy in one night for example—and he completely overreacts, throwing himself on the ground and becoming inconsolable. These overreactions may be more sporadic in your child than they were with Ryan, but they still can cause a lot of disruption and upset. Always remember that your child is going through major neurological, physiological, and emotional changes at this age—it's no one's fault. But you can help.

Sound Familiar?

- Do you feel like you're yelling too much at your child?
- Do you feel frustrated and out of ideas?
- Do you feel like other kids are much more easygoing than your child?
- Do you describe your child as "difficult"?
- Do you avoid certain people, places, and things for fear of how your child may react?
- Do you worry that your kid won't be able to sustain friendships?
- Do you feel like consequences are hard to figure out for your kid?
- If you are co-parenting, do you find yourselves disagreeing about how best to parent your child?
- Do you find yourself confused about whether your child has control over their behaviors?
- Have you asked yourself this question: "Is this normal?"

If this resonates with you, the good news is that this chapter includes a range of tools you can use that with practice and repetition can really help your child learn to manage his emotions, both the positive and negative ones.

PARADIGM SHIFT

Paradigm: The middle childhood years between kindergarten and middle school are a stable time when kids just settle down. The days of tantrums are thankfully behind us. If my child is moody, it's just his personality or he will grow out of it.

Shift: Children are going through a period of massive transition from six to twelve, and parents need to understand that this often affects mood, causing kids to act in confusing or upsetting ways. You can guide your child toward better emotional regulation, a skill he'll be able to use throughout adolescence and life. This starts with you.

Why Teaching Your Child to Regulate His Emotions at This Age Is So Important

Puberty is a particularly good time for children to learn how to regulate their emotions. During this phase, the hippocampus—the structure in the limbic system that is responsible for regulating emotions and memory—is generating thousands more cells than in adulthood. The theory is that it's an adaptive response to prepare a young animal to learn what it needs to in order to go out on its own. This means that kids in puberty have the brain capacity to easily absorb new ways of handling things. At the same time, the prefrontal cortex responsible for decision-making, problem-solving, planning, and regulating social behavior is also rewiring. This remodeling increases the brain's capacity for self-control. In other words, the more you can help your child to regulate his emotions at this age, the more those skills will be wired into his brain, with benefits that will last for a lifetime.

If you have a moody child, you may simply assume that he will outgrow these behaviors. After all, aren't all adolescents moody? Won't this behavior go away on its own when the brain and hormones settle down? Not necessarily. One of the first questions I asked Jaime and Greg was "What was Ryan like as a baby?" I wasn't surprised when Jaime answered that he was a "difficult" infant, hard to soothe. Studies show that temperament is generally a stable trait: some children are simply easier to deal with than others, and as parents with multiple children can attest, kids are born with one of three temperaments: easy, difficult, or cautious. When you realize and acknowledge that your child may have the kind of temperament that makes dealing with emotions challenging for him, you can tell yourself: "It isn't anything I've done... It's not my fault or anyone else's. I just have to find a way to work with *his* temperament."

I explained to Jaime and Greg that parenting Ryan was going to be different from parenting their other children. Once they could wrap their minds around the fact that Ryan simply had different needs from his brother and sister—and that one-size-fits-all parenting wasn't going to work—they were able to adjust their approach.

As I reassured Jaime and Greg, when a child learns to better regulate his moods, the payoff is enormous in the short and long term. Research has shown that self-regulation skills correlate with greater academic achievement, healthier friendships and relationships, less depression and anxiety, and improved social-emotional intelligence. The ability to self-regulate can also improve a child's impulse control, which allows for better judgment and decision-making by increasing the pause between the initial emotion and the reaction, and his awareness of his thoughts, feelings, and behavior. Regulation also correlates to improved cognitive flexibility, which allows kids to change the way they think about something. Children who can regulate are also easier on themselves—highly dysregulated people are often highly self-critical because they live with remorse and regret. Being more regulated allows kids to feel proud of themselves for how they handled situations and reduces self-criticism. It can help your child have a more positive affect and expression, improve his attention, and reduce his tendency to ruminate (overthink things). Incredibly, it can also help with improved working memory, which in turn improves cognitive efficiency, selective attention, and executive control.

Fortunately, lack of emotional regulation doesn't seem to be a fixed trait. With your help, your child can gain proficiency at this skill. Over time, he'll learn about the context of a situation (it's okay to yell at a football game but not in the middle of a test, for example) and have a broader range of experiences that will offer him multiple chances to learn and then apply this skill as he continues to grow up.

Understanding Your Child's Window of Tolerance

When I'm working with families where the child is emotionally dysregulated, one of the first things I'll talk about is the concept of "the window of tolerance." This was originally coined by Dr. Dan Siegel, a professor of psychiatry at the UCLA School of Medicine. According to Siegel, "Emotional Dysregulation is affective arousal that exceeds our window of tolerance. Each person's window of tolerance is constructed from biological sensitivities and their available regulation resources." In other words, when a child is operating within a situation that he can manage, he can deal with life, he can handle the everyday challenges thrown at him. When he's faced with something that he cannot manage, he cannot handle life's challenges, and he melts down, becomes unreasonable, and gets stuck. For example, children are often within their window of tolerance during the day when they're at school, and then when they get home and it's time to do homework, they're outside of it!

After introducing this concept of the window of tolerance to Ryan and his parents, I asked Ryan to draw parallel lines on the whiteboard I keep in my office to show me how large or small his window was for certain events. Then, I asked him to place certain people, places, and things that made him feel at ease inside the window and then have him place stressors or triggers outside the window. Ryan listed doing math games, playing with his dog, going to his grandma's, and goofing around with his younger sister as being inside his window. Outside of his window he listed going skiing with his family, reading, homework, going to sports practices, eating what his mom makes for dinner, cleaning up his room, taking a shower, brushing his teeth, and going away to summer camp. He added playing with friends right on the window line—

indicating that sometimes he found socializing easier and sometimes harder. There was a lot more that lay outside of his window than inside.

Kids who get easily frustrated or angry can have different windows of tolerance for different things. When Ryan was within this window, he was able to learn, play, and relate well to himself and others. However, if he moved outside of his window, he could become hyper-aroused. To be *hyper*-aroused means to be ready to fight or flee. It looks like anxiety, overwhelm, or aggression. Other children may become *hypo*-aroused, which means they freeze, and this manifests as shutting down, becoming depressed or withdrawn. Often children come home from school and take a giant nap at this age—they're outside of their window of tolerance and need to rest. Some children can have outsize positive emotions as well as becoming overly excited and unable to calm down—for instance, a child who wins a game may continue to jump up and down and brag long after it's appropriate to do so.

As a parent, thinking of your child as being either inside or outside of his window of tolerance can be really helpful. It gives you and your child a shared language that is less harsh or judgmental than questions like "Why do you always do this?" or "Why can't you just get with the program?" And it's simply more accurate. Remember these windows can open and close, so that your child who happily went to his grandparents last week may suddenly not want to go without a fight the next.

Luckily, there are ways that you can expand your child's window of tolerance and add activities, people, and places to it.

- Prepare for a situation that you know is outside your child's window of tolerance. If it's the first day of school and your child struggles with big transitions, you can make sure he walks into school with a friend.
- Adapt the environment when possible. If sensory issues bother your child, make sure the tags are cut out of his clothes or that his shoes are worn in. If your child struggles in noisy places, he can wear earplugs or noise-canceling headphones.
- Build in structure and consistency. Children who have a limited window of tolerance benefit when they know what to expect from each day. A regular morning and evening routine can help him cope with times when he's outside his window. Build in breaks if your child needs them, even with

activities he enjoys. You may have a super social child who loves going to his friends' birthday parties, but who melts down if he has to go to another social event after that. Building in time to go home and rest before moving on to another activity may be a game changer for a child like this.

- Take time to specifically praise your child when he is able to add something new inside his window—reflect on how he was able to successfully expand his window, and that you appreciate his effort. In this way, your child can learn that he's capable of doing new things, if you plan together in the right way.

The window of tolerance concept is easy for both parents and kids to relate to. In fact, college students who learned it in therapy with me as younger kids tell me they still use it in their day-to-day lives.

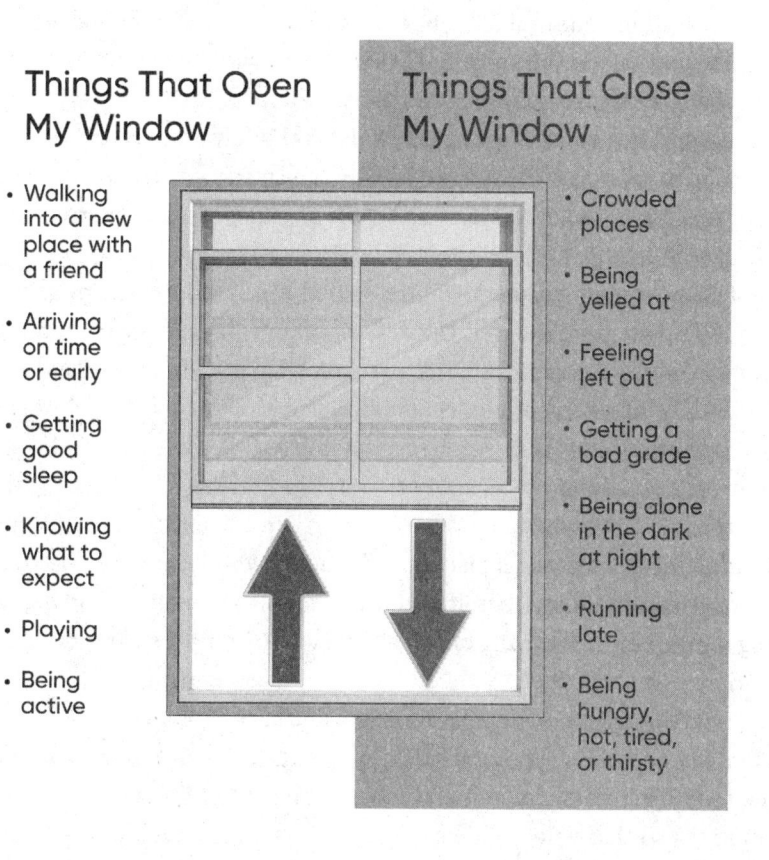

Things That Open My Window

- Walking into a new place with a friend
- Arriving on time or early
- Getting good sleep
- Knowing what to expect
- Playing
- Being active

Things That Close My Window

- Crowded places
- Being yelled at
- Feeling left out
- Getting a bad grade
- Being alone in the dark at night
- Running late
- Being hungry, hot, tired, or thirsty

Co-regulation and Self-regulation

Emotional regulation takes place when a child can effectively manage his feelings, thoughts, and actions. When a well-regulated child feels sad, he thinks to himself "I'm feeling sad," and he acts to seek the comfort he needs without taking it out on others or crying inconsolably. The ultimate goal is for your child to *self*-regulate—to respond to his emotional needs in a healthy way—but in order for that to happen, first you, the parent, will need to lead the way.

If you think about it, you've been helping your child to regulate since he was a baby. Back then, you gave him a pacifier or a special blanket to help him stop crying. You were calm enough to say, "The baby is upset, the pacifier should help soothe him, I'll give the baby the pacifier." And if that didn't work, you knew to try burping him, feeding him, rocking him. You tried out several tools in your tool belt until one worked. When your child grew to be a toddler, you gained the knowledge that if he was in the middle of a meltdown you could try to give him a hug and his blankie, and he would likely calm down pretty quickly. Eventually you experienced the reward of watching your crying child reaching for the blankie to calm himself down on his own. When this happened, your child had learned to *self-regulate*, but it all started with you, the parent, saying, "You're upset, let's get your blankie."

This term "self-regulation" was coined in the mid-1980s by the late Albert Bandura, an influential Canadian American psychologist and Stanford University professor. Since then, psychologists have built on Bandura's theory to develop different models of self-regulation. As a result, there are several definitions, but this is mine: self-regulation is the ability to be aware of your emotional and physical needs—and to find ways to meet those needs in healthy and productive ways. The problem for many parents during the middle childhood years is that it can feel more complicated to help your child to regulate at age nine than it was when he was an infant or toddler. Do you hug him? Distract him? Dig out the old blankie again? It's likely none of these tactics work any longer.

Even though your child has more advanced communication and cognitive skills than he did when he was a baby, the reality is he still needs you to set the tone. This means that you, the parent, need to calmly regulate your own emotions so that your child can do the same. This is called "co-regulation," and it's essential for helping children learn to *self*-regulate. It means you need to get your own feelings and thoughts under control first, so you can act from a place of calm in order to calm your child, which is often easier said than done when your child is angry, frustrated, and hurling accusations at you. Over time, if you can stay calm, your child will start to internalize the process of calming himself so he can do it without your help.

There's actually a lot of science behind the phenomenon of co-regulation. Studies show that when two people are together their brain oscillations can synchronize in a process called entrainment. When two or more brains are entrained with one another, co-regulation can happen. To put it in layman's terms, when your ten-year-old is yelling in frustration at you, you can either entrain with him by matching his mood and yelling back *or* you can do the opposite. You can take a deep breath, find a place of inner calm, and get him to entrain with your calm state of mind instead.

When it comes to entrainment or co-regulating with your child, often your most powerful tool is simply your presence. Sometimes saying nothing can be the best approach, helping him to calm down simply by standing close to him, using a gentle touch on the arm, or by making eye contact with him, adjusting your posture as you do it. Coming down closer to your child's height is often a nonverbal cue to the child that you want to meet him where he is, and that you're not a threat to him. This strategy works well for when you don't know what to say, or things have gotten very loud, or you can't reason with your child at that moment. Your calm, caring, patient demeanor actually has a neurological impact on the child's physiology and then his cognitive process—your demeanor affects his demeanor. When you do speak, adjust your tone of voice so that he knows that you want to help him not just scold him. And if you do yell, just correct yourself in the moment and focus on returning to a place of calm—a dysregulated adult cannot regulate a dysregulated child.

In an ideal situation, you can set the pattern or rhythm and tone for your child. That isn't always the case, even when you're a trained psychologist! I'll give you an example. My middle child regularly loses his homework, and as a person who is very organized, this drives me nuts. Over the years he's been in school, my reaction has been to get upset, saying things like "What is wrong with you, we created a folder for this, and you didn't even use it?" Or "Are you kidding me, *again* you lost your homework?" What I have learned from those mistakes is that I'm not going to shame my kid into remembering his homework. I get a lot further with him when I hold him accountable, create a plan, and help him, versus getting angry.

On a good day, if my son is frustrated because he lost his homework again, I can say softly, "I understand that losing your homework is very frustrating for you, you worked hard on it," while putting an arm around his shoulder, before working with him to make a plan so it doesn't happen again. Other times, if I've just come home from a busy day at work, his stress adds to mine and everyone ends up getting frustrated. When the stress is escalating, I can choose to model self-regulation for him. I take a deep breath, close my eyes, then go get a drink of water as a way of taking a break before returning to him in a better state of mind.

It's important to remember that although your child is no longer a toddler, he may not still be developed enough to consistently regulate his emotions without your help. This may also require you to acknowledge some of your own challenges around emotional regulation. I've come to realize that I react in this way to my son losing his homework because I worry he won't grow up to be an independent, self-sufficient young adult who can get through high school, much less college! Once I recognized this, I found I could control those thoughts, which freed me up to be responsive to him rather than just reacting. Remaining calm in the face of your child's outbursts can be especially difficult if you came from an emotionally confusing or volatile home where your own parents didn't give you any guidance around regulation. If growing up, your parents were prone to anger, then it may be especially triggering for you to see your child get angry. This could be a good time to reflect on your own childhood coping skills and adult ones. Which are healthy and helpful? Are there any that need some work?

Mindfulness

Angry, frustrated, or overwhelmed parents rarely have productive conversations with a kid. Before you can help your child calm down, you need to get yourself in a better place first, and mindfulness is one of the tools you can use to achieve this. In therapeutic terms, "mindfulness" simply means concentrating on the present moment. If any feelings, thoughts, or sensations intrude your mind, you can calmly acknowledge them and let them go, or put them to the side. Research has shown mindfulness is a powerful tool for stress reduction. Some researchers believe that by consistently activating our calming neurons, mindfulness practice can actually rewire our brains and make us less reactive thanks to the brain's neuroplasticity, its ability to form new connections in response to stimuli.

Understand that you may have to remove yourself from a situation to effectively practice mindful behavior. Let's say you and your child are in the middle of an interaction that you can tell is about to go sideways. Don't just walk away. Calmly tell him, "I need a minute to myself to think about what I want to say or do," and then practice a mindfulness strategy. Tell your child how long you think you'll need. You might also say something like "Maybe you can do something during this time that is helpful to you, too," or direct a younger child to a calming activity, which reinforces that you are taking a break because it will help you to reengage in a relationship with them, not because you don't care about them (which is sometimes how kids feel during an angry exchange with a parent).

Here are four mindfulness activities to try:

DIAPHRAGMATIC BREATHING, AKA DEEP BELLY BREATHING

Have you ever felt yourself kind of gasping when you are upset or stressed? There's a reason for that. Stress causes the *sympathetic* nervous system (the one that governs our ancient fight, flight, or freeze response) to activate—as if you were a hunter-gatherer facing a wildebeest rather than a parent trying to get their kid to do their homework. This releases the hormone adrenaline, which causes your heart to beat faster to pump more blood to important parts of your body, such as the muscles, that might be needed to fight or outrun the wildebeest. The rapid heart rate, along with an increase in blood pressure, may cause your chest to feel tight, making it difficult to breathe.

Belly breathing is one of the very best ways to counteract an adrenaline rush because it stimulates the *parasympathetic* nervous system—the one that helps us calm down, often referred to as the "rest and digest" system. It's my top recommendation because you can do this anywhere.

- Place one hand on your upper chest and the other just below your rib cage. This will allow you to feel your diaphragm move as you breathe.
- Breathe in slowly through your nose for four seconds so that your stomach moves out against your hand. The hand on your chest should remain as still as possible.
- Hold your breath for seven seconds.
- Tighten your stomach muscles, so that your stomach moves back in, as you exhale for eight seconds or longer through your mouth. The hand on your upper chest should remain as still as possible.

I suggest that you practice belly breathing every day, multiple times per day, not only because the practice will more easily come to you when you need it, but because studies suggest that consistent deep breathing exercises lower stress and promote relaxation.

Sometimes I feel like my clients are mentally rolling their eyes when I evangelize about breathing; they've heard it before. But it's extremely effective. I once worked with a forty-something-year-old man going through a divorce who needed help with the angry outbursts that had contributed to his marriage's demise and his strained relationship with his kids. I assigned him a breathing regimen to follow when he woke in the morning, when he got into the car, when he was enraged by someone else's behavior (usually while driving), and in the evening before bed. After a few weeks, he developed the ability to recognize when his anger was on the rise, and he was able to interrupt it with deep breathing and other mindfulness techniques he had been practicing. Within about six weeks, he reported improved relationships with his kids, his colleagues, fellow drivers, even his dog! He noticed that the kids were cautiously optimistic that dad wasn't as angry anymore, and he even got asked to go out to lunch with a group of colleagues, something that hadn't happened in the eight years since he'd first started the job.

INTENTION SETTING

If you've ever been to a yoga class, you might have been asked to set an intention at the beginning of the class. Your instructor may have encouraged you to focus on a thought that could help bring in your presence to your practice and, often, in life. Examples are: "I am grounded." "I am aware." "I am enough." You can do the same before stepping into your role as parent, say, after school or after work.

Research suggests that setting intentions that are specific, rather than vague, can help people achieve their goals. It's the difference between "I won't lose my temper tonight" and "I intend to engage with my family at dinner tonight with patience and understanding."

USING A MANTRA

You don't have to use a mantra during prayer or meditation for it to help regulate stress, but it's often a good idea. Repeating a mantra in response to stressful events, as well as practicing using it throughout the day to keep it top of mind, can actively lower stress levels.

I've used a mantra since the early months of parenthood when I was so exhausted that I wanted to cry along with my newborn daughter. I'm a person who loves her sleep, and I began to wonder how I would ever feel refreshed and energetic again. Then, one day, I decided to pick a mantra to help me reframe how tired I was. I settled on "attitude of gratitude" to remind me every morning that I was so fortunate to have a baby. Every day when my eyes opened to my new alarm—aka the baby monitor—I would say to myself "attitude of gratitude." Sometimes I would say it out loud. Sometimes I had to say it several times as I was walking to the nursery to shift my thoughts from how tired I was to how grateful I was to have this baby to care for. It was a game changer for me.

I stuck with this mantra even after the kids grew out of the sleep-stealing stage. To this day, every morning, I say "attitude of gratitude" to myself either before or as my feet hit the ground. It reminds me that this is what I always wanted: the career, the kids, the spouse, the house, the dog. And, if something goes wrong during the day, you might catch me taking a few deep breaths and whispering "attitude of gratitude" to myself.

MONOTASKING

Parents are often applauded for their abilities to multitask. And while this is a useful skill when it comes to, say, getting kids fed, dressed, and ready for school on time in the morning, it's actually counterproductive to mindfulness. Instead, try to monotask—which involves focusing on one task at a time—allowing you to be more present and less stressed, which is more conducive to self-regulation.

Not only is multitasking stressful, but research has shown that people who multitask are less productive and make more errors; our brains simply cannot pay high-level attention to more than one task. We also tend to overestimate our ability to multitask. In fact, some researchers believe the term "multitasking" is a misnomer.

The biggest culprit that robs our children of our attention is our phones. I know that phones allow us to be connected at all moments and you sometimes feel like you just have to respond to that work email or a friend's text. And I understand the dopamine rush that comes from scrolling or from solving the Wordle of the day. But besides missing out on the opportunity to talk to your kid or listen to their jokes, there are other reasons to stay off your phone and focus fully on them: A study of four hundred parents of kids ages five to twelve found that parents' use of phones negatively affected their children's emotional intelligence or EQ.[1] Phone use, especially when parents are distracted when with their kids, can lead to a lack of emotional responsiveness, which leads to their children not learning the cues and social-emotional exchanges needed to develop their EQ.

Tear and Repair

Remember—even if you do become reactive, shout, scream, and fail to model healthy regulation for your child, you can still turn that situation into a teachable moment. If you think of a relationship as a piece of fabric or a tie that binds two people together, you'll also know that this fabric can become ripped or torn. That's why I talk to parents about the concept of "tear and repair." A tear in a relationship is a psychological or emotional injury. With your child, it could look like yelling at your kid, speaking in all-or-nothing terms ("You always ruin our dinner" or "You never say thank you"), grabbing his arm a little too tightly when angry, calling him a name ("You're a spoiled brat"), cursing at him ("I'm so tired of this sh!t"), shaming him ("No one else was crying when they lost a game")—the list could go on and on. Our children can trigger us, and despite our intentions, we lose our patience, say things that we never thought we'd hear come out of our mouths, or repeat the dysfunctional way we were parented. I'm human; I have been there, too.

But what parents don't always realize is that we need to make a repair when we have caused a tear. Sometimes that takes the form of an apology: a sincere, no-buts-or-excuses acceptance of responsibility. Acknowledge what has happened: "I had a really tough day, and I lost my patience with you." Then you can apologize, "I'm sorry for yelling and not listening to you. I'll keep working on being a better listener and taking deep breaths when I feel myself getting upset." When you do this (with no buts or excuses) you're teaching your child: we all make mistakes; our job is to learn from our mistakes and practice what we learn the next time a challenging situation arises. Sometimes it's a moment of vulnerability, admitting you were scared about something and overreacted, adding that you'll work on managing your fear responses. Sometimes, it's recognizing your child for how he kept calm while you lost your cool and even asking him how he was able to do that. Modeling "tear and repair" can reinforce that mistakes or setbacks are to be expected in life, especially while learning new things. It tells your child, "I am in relationship with you; when one of us struggles we can move through it together." Repairing models a competency you want your child to achieve: the ability to handle tough conversations, forgive another person, and reconnect after a rupture.

The repair skill will help you to create your own paradigm shift, from "I am a terrible parent. I yell at my kids too much" to "I am a parent committed to learning every day. I've made some mistakes that have caused tears in our relationships, and I am going to work on repairing them and preventing ruptures in the future." This will also help your child establish trust in your relationship, so he learns to trust himself and eventually others in friendship, intimacy, and love.

Ask Yourself "Who Holds the Energy Here?"

When it comes to dealing with your child's moods and reactions, I want you to imagine you're wearing a tool belt. You'll need to put on this tool belt every morning: here's where you keep your hammer, your wrench, your measuring tape—just the basics. What we're going to do together is to figure out which are the tools that are most helpful for you and your child.

Some of my favorite parenting tools take the form of questions you can ask yourself whenever your child is upset. One of these questions is "Who holds the energy here?" or "Who's in charge here?" If the answer is "My child holds the power" and you want to be the one in control, the first thing you need to do is get into a regulated state, so that your state of calm is stronger than your child's state of upset. Remember, the most important person in the room when it comes to setting the mood is *you*, the parent. That's why it's so important to put on your own oxygen mask first, take that deep breath, get that glass of water, and *then* assess what your child needs. It may sound idealistic at first, but with practice, it becomes easier and more natural to take hold of the energy in the room, which in turn will help your child to calm down. And over time, your child will follow your lead, learning that when he's stressed or upset, he has the power to calm himself, even if you're not there.

Figuring Out What Your Child Really Needs: Attunement

In this chapter, we've been focusing on your child's emotional regulation—and your own state of calm to help your child get to a place where he can begin to regulate his own emotions. In order for this to happen, you need to figure out what your child really needs and what triggers him. This means you need to practice attunement.

Attunement refers to the ability of one person to tune into the needs of another. Marriage expert John Gottman came up with this acronym that explains its elements:

Attention
Turn Toward
Understand
Non-defensively listen
Empathize

When you tune in to and connect with your child's needs, it fosters a sense of security and emotional well-being in your child. Another way I sometimes refer to this is emotional synchronicity. When you can read and respond to your child's needs, he responds back to you with a sense of security and love.

Attunement is one of the most important skills in your parenting tool belt, and it's one you can use for a lifetime. But it takes work because it demands not only self-awareness ("What am I doing?" "How am I feeling?" "Do I know what I am saying?") but also the ability to be aware of your child's mood ("What are they doing?" "How do they feel?" "Does this look like a good time to be discussing an issue?")

Attunement will be familiar to you from back in the day when you first became a parent. Back then, you looked at your baby, your baby smiled, you smiled too. When your toddler dropped a toy, you attuned to him by saying, "Uh-oh! Let's pick it up." Attunement is meeting your child where he's at and tuning in to what he feels or needs. It involves reading the room and then changing your energy to match what's happening. For some people, attunement comes naturally; for others it can take a lot more practice.

The opposite of attunement is misattunement: it's when you don't fully understand your child's needs, you miss signals, or you have trouble reading your child's nonverbal cues. I once had a family session where the father laughed when his child told him that she tripped while getting up onstage at school, rather than "tuning in to" the fact that his daughter didn't think it was funny at all but felt horribly embarrassed instead. This parent later shared that he was trying to make light of the moment so as to not make a big deal of it. The problem with this strategy was that his child experienced him as insensitive and uncaring, even if he was trying to be lighthearted in order to make her feel better.

Your child's needs are not always going to be so easy to read as when he was younger, but he's still looking to you for cues about how to deal with life's daily problems. There's no trick to attunement. Instead, it requires empathy, sensitivity, and willingness to engage in trial and error.

Different emotional states need different kinds of attunement. When your kid comes home from school feeling sad and dejected because he got into an argument with a friend, attuning to him would mean adjusting your tone and body language to his. You're not going to approach him with high energy and a smile. Instead, you can sit down next to him and lean toward him, saying, "I can see you're really upset about something." If your child is in a rage about something that happened with a sibling, using a soft, neutral tone can make things worse. Instead, you can meet him at a higher vibration by using an intense, emphatic voice as you say, "Whoa, buddy, I can see you're upset, I'm right here with you."

Maybe your kid will benefit from a sympathetic touch on the arm or shoulder. Maybe he needs you to make eye contact with him, or for you to be super quiet so that you're just matching him with your presence. Maybe he wants you to make a joke that you know he will enjoy or provide him with some other kind of distraction. You might simply acknowledge the problem and tell your child you're committed to brainstorming solutions with him. You could just decide to say, "That sucks, I'm so sorry." Whichever way you choose to attune to your child, he will get the message loud and clear that he's understood and you're there for him.

Attunement is especially important when parents and children get home from school, when you've been away from each other for a period of time, and when you're most likely to be misattuned. For example, you come in from work and the babysitter tells you that your eldest is upset with her because she said no to extra cookies, but he's playing on the iPad, and he's starting to calm down. Remember, in this moment, you're entering your child's space and that your first step should be attuning to him. But how can you do this if you haven't been with him all day? Instead of coming in guns blazing, telling him to get off the screen so you can discuss what happened with the sitter, quietly go and sit next to him. Trust that if you don't force the conversation, if you allow it to happen in your child's time, it will come. Eventually, he may look up and tell you, "Ellie made me so mad today," and then you can begin. By attuning to your child as the first step, meeting him where he is, you stand a much better chance of finding out what's really going on with him and addressing the issue. After you've made that connection, you can even begin to brainstorm next steps with your child. "What do you think you need to say or do for Ellie now that you are calm?"

Remember that your response will also need to be context dependent. In some situations, the best response may be for you to step away, giving your child some privacy so he can cry it out. (This works well when you aren't pressured for time.) Sometimes you may want to give your child a weighted blanket to calm him down. (This works well at home where you have access to it.) You'll need a variety of tools as what works in one situation may not work as well in another.

Attunement can look like leaning in or stepping back. Talking or silence. Distraction or focus. It's a relationship art that can be hard to practice when we ourselves are dysregulated because we are tired, hungry, or stressed. But as with any art, the more you practice it, the more naturally it will come.

And if you are ever really trying and your kid doesn't seem to be responding, say to them, "I have tried a couple things that I thought would be helpful, but they don't seem to be helping right now. Do you have any tips for me?" Showing humility doesn't weaken you as a parent. It strengthens trust in your relationship, and kids love to teach their parents things; it's a win-win.

If you're reading this and you're thinking, "Oh no! I'm not sure how good I've been at this attunement thing!" It's okay. Remember a child's brain is still malleable at this age. There's plenty of time to work on this.

Active Listening

One of the biggest complaints kids share with me is "My parents just don't listen . . ." A child's confidence, self-esteem, and ability to manage stress are heavily affected by the way he was taught to communicate. If he's often criticized and corrected he will feel like everything he does is wrong and that he is a failure. On the other hand, a child who's being raised by someone who listens and who focuses on what he's really saying will have much better communication skills of his own.

It's not enough to just hear the words coming from your child, you need to be an active listener. Here are some helpful tips that will sound like basic communication skills, but they're actually quite challenging for many parents to consistently implement.

1. Make time to talk with your child on a daily basis, encouraging him to share his thoughts and feelings. This conversation needs to go beyond "Did you do your homework?" or "How was your day?" You need to be focused solely on your child (put your phone away) and remain present even if the conversation gets long or difficult. Don't correct small things and don't finish his sentences.
2. Assume an active listening position. Come down to your child's level. Sit close to him. Show him through your body language that he has your whole attention.
3. Give your child options for how he wants you to respond. You can ask something like "What would be most helpful from me right now? Do you want me to just listen, or do you want to hear my suggestion, or do you want to hear what I think?"
4. Don't try to solve your child's problems. I understand you may want to fix things. That's only natural for parents, and it's why your instinct will be to listen to a little bit of the situation and then jump in with solutions. Your priority is fixing whatever you consider wrong—whether it's your child's behavior or their hurt feelings. But some kids *hate* the problem-solving approach; for them, the priority is being heard and acknowledged.

When you make a point of regularly practicing active listening with your child, this will help you in everyday encounters with your kid and in your other relationships too.

Learn to Verbally Validate Your Child

Children who are dysregulated like Ryan will usually tell me that they don't feel heard or understood by others. They'll report that their parents say things to them like "Stop making such a big deal out of nothing" or "Just stop crying." Although parents often mean well when they say these things—hoping that their words will help children to better regulate—they wind up dismissing their child's feelings, making the child feel unimportant. In psychology, we use the term "psychological invalidation" to describe what happens when someone rejects, dismisses, or minimizes someone else's thoughts, feelings, or experience, thereby communicating that these thoughts, feelings, or experiences are not real or worthy. This can be through judgment ("You shouldn't be this upset over this") or blame ("If you just would have listened to me this wouldn't have happened"). Invalidation can take the form of you, the parent, walking away or ignoring a child when he's upset or getting so dysregulated that you start to match the emotional intensity of your child, which usually results in two highly upset people with few to no resources in that moment to come up with a solution.

The good news is that research on dysregulation suggests that kids who have a hard time regulating their emotions respond well to validation. If children feel listened to and respected, they tend to be able to return to a state of calm more easily. Validation leads to a more secure relationship between parent and child and reduces the need for your child to get as intense as usual because he feels heard and understood. To be clear, validation is not the same as agreeing. Here's an example of what I mean:

Your child comes home from school in tears, telling you, "Everyone hates me." Every parent has a hard time seeing a child who is upset or unhappy. Every parent wants to make their child feel better. Your instinct might be to respond, "Of course everyone loves you! You have so many friends!" But that reaction can quickly backfire on you—and here's why.

First, your child won't believe you. Of course, you think he's popular and talented and beautiful: you're his parent! Second, by disagreeing with him, you've confused him, because at that moment, he genuinely feels as if everyone hates him. And third, by contradicting him, it will seem to him as if you're dismissing his pain—you've invalidated him.

Helping to develop a child's self-regulation means accepting his thoughts and feelings, regardless of how much you may disagree with them. When I work with parents, I teach them that the best way to respond in a way that validates a child's emotion is to actively listen, add verbal validation, plus empathy, plus curiosity (if you have a clarifying question), plus a bridge statement to encourage your child to process the feeling. It might go like this:

Child: Everyone hates me.

Parent: (in active listening position, starts out by validating) Oh, you feel like nobody likes you . . .

Child: Yeah. Today no one wanted to be my science partner.

Parent: (empathizing) It can hurt our feelings to feel left out.

Child: I don't understand why no one picked me.

Parent: (curiosity) I wonder . . .

And then hold space. If the child doesn't fill in, you can add something like "If there weren't enough people for everyone to have a partner."

Child: Yeah, I was the only one left.

Parent: (bridge statement) I wish . . . I could help your hurt feelings. I hear . . . how hard that was for you. I know how much you care about your friendships.

By resisting the urge to point out that this experience hardly means that everyone hates him, you have made your child feel listened to, understood, and capable of handling difficult feelings. By repeating out loud what he's telling you—in essence, simply serving as a mirror for him—you've allowed your child the space to discover how he's really feeling. Maybe by the end of this conversation your child has realized it's not that everyone hates him but that it might be a good idea to try to make other friends in this particular class.

Being Responsive vs. Reactive

A reactive parent doesn't stop and think before acting. Instead, this parent reacts impulsively, and often with high emotion. Have you ever given in to your child, despite knowing that's not what's best for them? Have you ever escalated when your child is escalating and gotten louder when your child was getting loud? To practice being a *responsive* parent rather than a reactive one, you need to be able to take a breath, give yourself time to consider what is best for your child, and not get caught up in high emotions. Take time to try and understand what's going on with your child. Think about what your child needs in the moment and also be aware of how you are feeling (frustrated, angry, tired, annoyed). You will still have typical human emotions; you will just know how to control them so you can more effectively respond to your child with clarity and confidence.

> ### Containment
>
> When it comes to helping your child regulate his emotions, the practice of containment is one of the most useful tools in your parenting toolbelt. Containment means "holding space" for your child's big emotions. Every single child has an unspoken need for you to do this. He can't articulate this need, but I promise you, this is what he wants. He doesn't want to be judged or lectured or fought with when he's experiencing emotions that are tough for him to control; he wants to be emotionally contained. So how do you do this?
>
> Think back to when he was a toddler having a tantrum. Your instinct as a parent was to hold him—to contain him—as he cried, screamed, and kicked. Fast-forward to middle childhood. Your child is going through tremendous physical and neurological changes. At this age, he still needs to be held, but now it's in a new way. An emotional way. Being an emotional container means accepting your child for who he is, sticking with him through his moods and challenges, and saying things that are supportive and helpful, not inflammatory. It means staying present and calm and not taking things personally. When you contain in this way, you're telling your child, "I am with you. I've got you. I accept all the parts of you; even the hard, messy, hurtful ones. I love you unconditionally and I am not going away. You're not alone. You're not too much for me, I can handle this, even as I am learning how to as we grow together."
>
> Remember, at this age, your child is likely feeling overwhelmed and confused by his emotions on a daily basis. He's spending a lot of time wishing things were different; and sometimes even feeling like he hates the way he behaves. If you can offer him this kind of containment for his emotions, as time goes on, he'll become more and more capable of

> understanding himself and what he's feeling. Accepting him as he is (not as you wish he was, or as he used to be) will model how he can do this for himself. He'll learn to be gentle with himself because patience and understanding were modeled for him. With consistency, this eventually leads to a greater ability to self-regulate.

Avoid Blaming or Shaming: How to Conceptualize Challenging Situations for Your Child

Research has shown that the way a parent conceptualizes challenging situations for a child can have lifelong implications on his mental health. What do I mean by "conceptualizing challenging situations"? Let's use an example: your child loses his temper and hurts his sister's feelings. How you conceptualize these events for him is key. If you say, "Stop being horrible to your sister, you can see she's upset! Why do you always do this with her? It's mean and I don't like it!" then you're blaming and shaming your child without giving him context for his behavior. As a result, he's getting the message: "I hurt my sister's feelings, I always do this, therefore I'm a bad person." In psychology, this is called "attributional bias." You're blaming your child's behavior on his *character* rather than the *context*. When you put the emphasis on traits rather than circumstances in this way, your child will likely internalize your criticism and take it personally, and this can negatively affect the belief patterns he will have about himself in the future.

Instead, you can say: "Hey buddy, let's take a time-out. You seem cranky today. Do you think you're tired because you went to bed late last night and that's why you're acting mean to your sister? Let's go and say sorry to her now and try to go to bed earlier tonight." In this scenario, you're sending him the message that there's a reason for his behavior, and that you are ready to work with him on modifying it and repairing the situation with his sister. Over time, this kind of healthy contextualization will positively impact his belief patterns and his ability to self-regulate.

Ask Yourself: Love or Fear?

Modern life is extremely busy. It can be hard to carve out time in your day to recap and reflect on your parenting decisions. But when you pause and think about the challenges you faced with your child and how you reacted or responded, you're gathering important information you can use in the days ahead. Whether you do this on your own, or talk about it with your partner or a friend, take a minute or two to pause and think about the day before bedtime. As you do this, ask yourself, "Was I acting out of love or fear today?"

I often ask parents this fundamental question: "Which emotion were you coming from: love or fear?" I borrowed the concept from decades of research by Elisabeth Kübler-Ross and David Kessler, experts on death and dying. They note that "deep down, there are only two emotions: love and fear. All positive emotions come from love, all negative emotions from fear. From love flows happiness, contentment, peace, and joy. From fear comes anger, hate, anxiety, and guilt."

Asking this question is one of the single greatest tools to help you respond versus react to your children, especially while your child is struggling. Stop and ask yourself, "Do I want to come from a place of love or fear?" This can really shift your mindset and the outcome.

To give an example: you're dropping a child off at a new friend's house but suddenly he doesn't want to go.

Fear response: If you are working from the emotion of fear, you might be feeling annoyed, ashamed that your child is acting this way, worried that the other kid's parents will think poorly of you and your child. As a result, you might say to your child, "You need to learn how to make new friends. Just get out of the car and walk inside, it will be fine."

Love response: If you are working from a place of love, you might be feeling concern, but also acceptance and support and might say, "I can see that going to a new friend's house is scary to you, let me help you."

> In both these examples, the parent wants the same thing for the child (to work through his worries and enjoy himself on a playdate). But one approach comes from a place of support, patience, and belief that the child can learn to handle the situation. The other tends to come from a place of fear mixed with a parent's baggage. This parent is thinking: "I used to be like this as a kid and I will be damned if my kid is going to be paralyzed with fear. He won't get invited back or have any friends if he doesn't just figure out how to just get in there and do it. What will this mom think of me? I have been sitting outside of their house for ten minutes, they must be wondering what is going on . . ."

Looking Ahead

A few short years from now your child will be a teenager and, in all likelihood, will be dealing with higher-stake situations. He'll find himself in all kinds of new circumstances, either in his social life or in the online world, that confuse or concern him. When you take the time to establish consistent communication with your six- to twelve-year-old, this means there's a routine and predictability to your connection, which makes it easier for him to approach you in the future when he needs a listening ear or guidance. If you lay the groundwork now, you'll reap the benefits later on when he comes to you to talk about how to ask someone on a date or to admit that he has had too much to drink and can't drive home.

In a Nutshell

When it comes to helping your child regulate his emotions, there are simple techniques that you, the parent, can implement that will have a major impact on your child. When you follow these principles, you're going to find that your child becomes much more flexible, and more likely to follow any rules or boundaries you set for him.

You can:

- Co-regulate
- Ask yourself "Who holds the energy here?"
- Practice attunement
- Practice containment
- Validate your child verbally
- Practice conceptualizing challenges for your child in a healthy way
- Ask yourself, Am I acting from a place of love or fear?

By doing so, you're actively modeling for your child how to manage his emotions. Slowly, over time, if you can consistently attune to your child, you'll start to see him mirroring your behavior. He'll begin problem-solving instead of panicking and taking a deep breath instead of freaking out.

This work is hard. It takes time and focus, but I believe this is the road map for a brighter future for any child. So many parents are focused on their child's academics, but emotional skills are just as, if not more, crucial to his future success, allowing him to have healthy relationships and protecting him against some of the pitfalls of adolescence and young adulthood such as anxiety and depression. These emotional skills will enable him to thrive academically, too. In other words, this work is worth it.

CHAPTER 4

The Unexpected Emotional Ups and Downs of Middle Childhood

What Kids Can Do

Oh, my gosh! I'm Anxiety. Where can I put my stuff?

—Anxiety, from Disney Pixar's *Inside Out 2*

In the last chapter, you learned about how to regulate your emotions as a parent in order to forge a healthy relationship with your child. In this chapter, we're going to focus on regulation skills for *your child*: empowering him to regulate his emotions, even when you're not around.

You'll remember nine-year-old Ryan and his parents Jaime and Greg whom you met in the last chapter. Even if your child isn't chronically dysregulated like Ryan, you're still going to deal with moodiness, outbursts, whining, and meltdowns during middle childhood. Children who struggle to regulate their emotions can be psychologically inflexible, they can be rigid in their thoughts and routines, and they can have low frustration tolerance. I've seen many well-meaning, thoughtful parents driven to the edge by children who only want to do things their own way, and whose emotions can quickly escalate when that doesn't happen.

After Jaime and Greg realized the importance of modeling emotional regulation for Ryan, they both made a concerted effort to reduce yelling and threatening. Jaime recognized that in the moment when she felt frustrated and upset with Ryan, she could take a "parent time-out" to calm herself down first so she could effectively co-regulate with her child. When Ryan was having a meltdown, Jaime's instinct was to send him to his room in the hope he would cool off, but we discovered that what helped Ryan the most was having an energy outlet. Dad served as a great distractor in this respect—taking Ryan outside to throw a ball around or to do tricks on his scooter. When Dad was away working, Jaime did the same. By tuning in, both parents were able to figure out what Ryan needed to regulate rather than escalate.

While working closely with Ryan's parents, I was also meeting with Ryan one-on-one. My goal was to get Ryan to a point where he could manage his emotions whether he was responding to internal stimuli ("I'm hungry," "I think I'm dumb," "I feel nervous that the teacher is going to call on me," "The last time I played over there that kid kicked me") or external stimuli ("It's loud in the cafeteria," "It smells bad in the bathroom," "It's too bright in my classroom," "The kid next to me won't stop tapping his pencil").

Ryan learned:

1. How to be a feelings detective—to correctly identify his emotions and feelings.
2. How to name it—naming whatever had triggered these feelings (what made him sad/mad/upset) and put words to the feeling. We call it "name it to tame it."
3. How to be mindful—learning to predict, prevent, and manage these feelings in the moment.

As I got to know Ryan better, I discovered he was an incredibly creative, thoughtful kid, who often felt out of control and became upset when he couldn't get his way—mainly because he wanted to feel a greater sense of control. By giving Ryan a variety of techniques he could use whenever he felt triggered, he was able to recognize he was not helpless and instead got to experience pride for how he dealt with certain situations. At times, he was even able to identify what might trigger him and plan for it, which further helped him handle his big feelings.

Many parents with children this age assume that kids should know how to calm themselves on their own by now. Parents often question why their kid, "hasn't grown out of this behavior yet." They're baffled by why their child seems like they have regular tantrums and meltdowns. It's important to remember that even when kids are intermittently dysregulated, they're still learning how to deal with the internal (hormones and brain changes) and external (peers and school expectations) stressors that are mounting around them. Meanwhile, kids who are more chronically dysregulated are likely to be wired this way due to a host of different factors such as temperament, early life experiences, parenting styles, genetics, neurological functioning, family history, sleep habits, comorbid physical or mental conditions, or a trauma history.

Regardless of the reasons why your child may experience emotional dysregulation, he'll benefit from learning skills that will help him to manage stress in puberty, adolescence, and adulthood. Children need to be systematically *taught* how to identify their feelings and calm their own bodies. It doesn't always happen naturally. Teaching them how to do these things may take a little while, but if you stick with it, I promise it will pay off.

Sound Familiar?

- Does your kid seem irritable for no reason?
- Do you sometimes feel like you're walking on eggshells around your kid?
- Do you feel like your child seems too old to be having tantrums? Did you think you were past this stage?
- Does your kid struggle with transitions and at mealtimes?
- Is your kid particularly whiny? Does he seem to be more sensitive than other kids? Does your child cry and complain easily?
- When your child is upset, do they flop or kick things or throw things?
- Does your kid verbally insult you? When your child is upset, do they act or say things in a way that's totally different from the way they are at other times?
- Does your child complain about things like certain material, tags, or seams, and do they only like to wear certain clothes?
- Is your kid able to keep it together at school but then comes home and falls apart?
- Do you avoid certain places or people because your child's behavior is context dependent?

> **PARADIGM SHIFT**
>
> **Paradigm:** My child will grow out of the moodiness, emotional outbursts, and whining when he gets older and he's through puberty.
>
> **Shift:** Middle childhood is the perfect time to help my child gain the tools he needs to manage, not just grow into, emotions. If I can teach him to understand emotions now, I'll have given him skills he needs for the rest of his lifetime.

Tools for Kids

THE FEELINGS DETECTIVE: IDENTIFYING EMOTIONS

The first step in helping your child to regulate his emotions is to give him the words to correctly name and identify them. When you give your child a vocabulary for his feelings and emotions, you also give him a way to understand them, because if you can't name a feeling, you can't identify it, much less manage it in a productive way. Although in academia, there's differing opinions on how many primary emotions we have, professor and renowned psychologist Dr. Paul Ekman—who has spent his lifetime studying emotions—has settled on six: joy, sadness, fear, anger, disgust, and surprise. Within those emotions, however, there is a whole spectrum of words that are at our disposal to describe how we feel: everything from "annoyed" and "frustrated" to "confused" and "ecstatic." The way I like to explain it to kids is that feelings are complicated. If they were simple, we'd only have a few emojis. Instead, there are at least ten emojis for sadness alone: anguished face, crying face, sad but relieved face, pensive face, worried face, loudly crying face, slightly frowning face, face holding back tears, frowning face, and a face with a teardrop. I tell kids I want their feelings vocabulary to be as wide as their phone's emojis. ☺

Often, children who are emotionally dysregulated have a hard time identifying and talking about how they're feeling. As a therapist, I must get creative, becoming a kind of feelings detective, and asking the child to join me in figuring out the mystery. In my office, I have a poster on the wall with thirty illustrations of different facial expressions with the names of the corresponding emotions underneath each one. If I want a child to open up to me, I'll just point at the poster and ask, "How are you feeling right now?" Sometimes the child picks the word, and sometimes he points to the picture. Often, children will tell me they don't know what the word means but that the picture is how they feel. I also have a box of stuffed emoji faces with the feeling words written on them. This was Ryan's preferred way to open up to me. I'd ask him, "How was your week, Ryan?" And then he would throw me a stuffed emoji from the box to answer my question. Then I'd throw him another emoji and ask, "When was the last time you felt this way?" And we'd throw the emojis back and forth.

Between the ages of six and nine in particular, you have a golden opportunity to teach the language of emotions to your child. Children in the earlier part of middle childhood tend to be more open about their emotions than when they get older and begin to shut you out. Older kids have a greater need for privacy and won't always want to talk about how someone at school hurt their feelings or how they're embarrassed about a teacher who criticized them. With each passing year, their interest in talking it out with you will go down and you'll have to get more creative and flexible to engage them to open up.

Even if your child does shut you out, it's important not to be put off. Many children struggle to answer questions such as "How was your day?" or "How did that make you feel?" and so as a parent, you'll have to get creative. Don't be afraid to be silly and playful. You don't have to come up with anything particularly elaborate; you just need to be curious.

Here are some ideas:

- Use emotional literacy tools. There are all kinds of products available to help you expand your child's emotional vocabulary, including magnets, flash cards, and stickers. You could put up an emoji poster on your refrigerator and ask your child to point at it to help him answer the question "How did that make you feel?" Or use flashcards with emojis on them to do the same. For younger kids, reading books together where characters experience different feelings and emotions can also be a good prompt for a discussion about how they feel. For older kids, paying attention to the books they read independently can help you spark up conversations too.
- Play a guessing game with your child. "I know how you're feeling, you're absolutely over*joyed* that the babysitter came to pick you up

from school instead of Dad—am I right?" You can play a "hot" or "cold" game, where you guess how your child was feeling in a certain situation before asking, "Am I hot or cold?" Remember to avoid interrogating your child; be light and use a joking tone when appropriate. Use a range of "feelings" words while you're guessing, which he can file away for later use.

- Ask your child to draw it out. You can journal together in a notebook by asking questions and then drawing the answers. At this age, nonverbal processing is just as valuable as verbal processing. If your child is younger, you can also put on music and dance around with your kid, asking him to show you how he feels with his movements.
- Wait until bedtime to chat with your child when he may let his guard down and be more open to sharing with you. And as parents of teens will attest, even the sulkiest adolescent will often open up when you're driving around sitting next to one another in the car.
- Be curious about your child's interests, music tastes, favorite TV shows, movies, podcasts—all of these can provide a great entry point into talking about your child's feelings and social situations. Take a few minutes to watch the video or listen to the podcast: your kid will be pleased that you did it and you will have deposited goodwill in the bank.
- If your kid *really* doesn't want to talk to you about how he's feeling, respect that. You can say, "You don't have to tell me, I just want you to know that I'm here for you." Patience is important—you can let it be for a night or day, then come back and revisit the subject.
- When you can see your child is upset and you're trying to figure out what happened, it's best not to ask the question "What happened?" Instead, you can ask your child to tell you the story of his day. Be curious. Ask him to recount what was happening *before* he got upset, what happened *during*, and what happened *after*. In this way, you'll be able to get a lot more information out of him about what happened and why.
- Many school districts are starting to incorporate social-emotional learning into their curriculums.[1] Ask your child's teacher if they have a social-emotional curriculum. If they do, look at the lessons with your child and talk them through. Use this as an opportunity to let your child teach you, learning with your child as you go. It's reinforcing for a kid's learning if you can use the same language he's hearing at school.

How Are You Feeling?

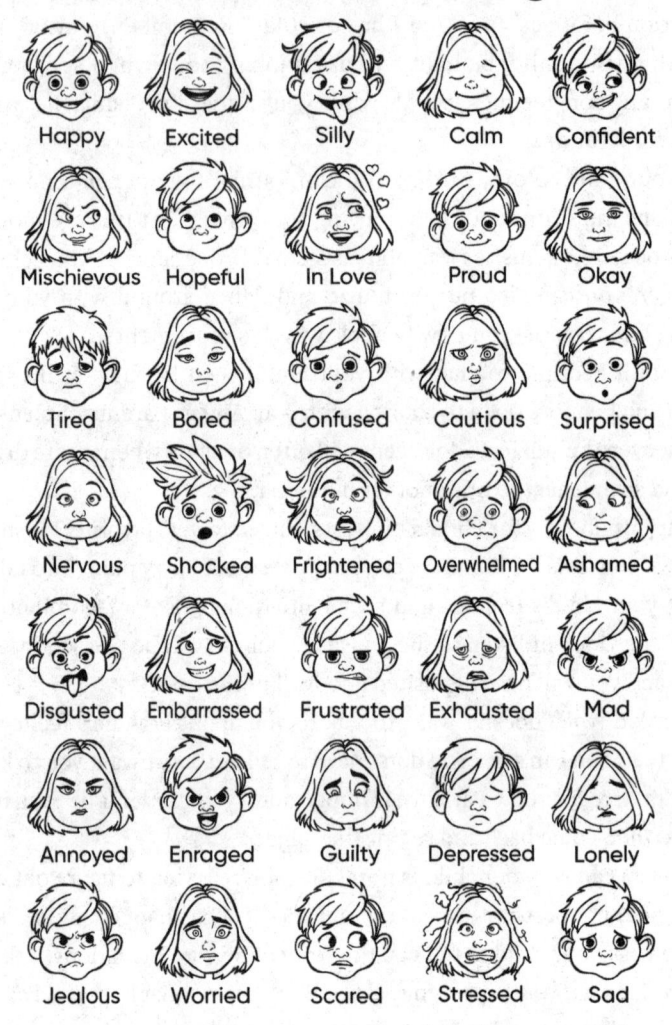

Happy	Excited	Silly	Calm	Confident
Mischievous	Hopeful	In Love	Proud	Okay
Tired	Bored	Confused	Cautious	Surprised
Nervous	Shocked	Frightened	Overwhelmed	Ashamed
Disgusted	Embarrassed	Frustrated	Exhausted	Mad
Annoyed	Enraged	Guilty	Depressed	Lonely
Jealous	Worried	Scared	Stressed	Sad

Don't get upset if you're met with silence. Remember that if you ask your child, "How are you feeling?" and he doesn't respond, this doesn't mean you've failed to get him to open up. In fact, silence can be a good sign. After all, if your kid immediately tells you, "I don't want to talk to you!" then it's unlikely he's going to share his innermost feelings with you. If the response is nothing, then take a breath and wait. Your child will talk to you in time.

Identifying Triggers, Proactive Planning, and Alternative Solutions

When I'm working with kids like Ryan on emotional regulation, I'll often tell them, "You know, things can feel out of your control sometimes—but there are probably a lot more things you can predict will make you feel upset or angry than you might think." Then I ask the child to tell me some situations that make him upset or angry whether at school or at home. He might say, "I hate it when my parents tell me to get off my video game—that makes me mad." Or "I get upset every time I have to go on the school bus and my parents can't drive me to school." Kids tend to know most of their triggers well and can often come up with a list for me. The reason we make a list together is so that the child has an awareness of the things that trigger him and also so the transitions going on inside and around him suddenly don't feel so scary.

Once the child has identified what makes him feel a certain way, we can start to proactively plan around these events. For example, you may have a child who is triggered by the transition back to school on Monday morning. He refuses to get out of bed, he cries and complains at having to get dressed, he won't put his lunch and water bottle in his backpack. The first step is to work with your child on identifying this trigger ahead of time.

"Hey kiddo," you can say to him on Sunday evening. "Tomorrow morning you're back to school. I know sometimes you get really grumpy on Monday mornings. Remember last week? You wouldn't get out of bed on time, so you missed the bus and I had to drive you. And when you got to the classroom you were really upset. You told me you don't like going into class when you feel that way. So what could we do differently tomorrow morning?"

And then you can invite your child to help you figure out a better way. Ask him to brainstorm with you, walking through the Monday morning process and figuring out a plan for what will happen. Be intentional—ask your child for his ideas, give him as much say as possible over how things get done. "Do you want to pack your backpack tonight or in the morning? Do you want to wear the white sneakers or the black sneakers tomorrow? Do you want to walk to the bus alone or with the other kids?" What you're doing is planning proactively so that Monday mornings suddenly feel more within his control.

The fact is that even after you've proactively planned with your child, he's not necessarily going to pop out of bed on Monday morning and cheerfully get ready for school on time. But when he starts whining because he can't find his black sneakers, you can say to him, "Remember? Last night you said you wanted to wear the black ones. That's why your black sneakers are at the door." By doing this, you're making things feel more predictable for your child who feels out of control.

When your child follows some element of the plan you've laid out together, you can specifically reinforce that behavior: "I see you laid out your black sneakers for school tomorrow. Let's see if that makes things easier in the morning." This sends him the message that he's on the right track. Over time, he will learn to proactively plan even without your prompting.

Another key technique that you can work on with your child is what I call "alternative solutions." Again, as with proactive planning, you're inviting your child to brainstorm with you. Let's say the morning routine doesn't go as well as you'd hoped, and your child ends up yelling at you because of something neither of you had predicted—you didn't hear him tell you that he wanted pancakes instead of waffles. When he gets home from school later in the day you can revisit this. You can say, "I know you were mad and frustrated with me this morning because I didn't hear you when you said you wanted pancakes. You yelled at me that I never listen to you. It's true that sometimes when I'm busy I get distracted. But what's another way you could have dealt with that without yelling at me?"

And then the two of you can brainstorm alternatives and even role-play the solutions you come up with:

"I could use my words. I could tell you that I'm upset and frustrated because you're not listening."

"I could have put my own waffles in the toaster, and you could have put the pancakes in the freezer for another time."

"I could have not said anything and just eaten the pancakes."

When you do this for your child, you're teaching him to be what I call a "solution seeker." Early on in my career, I was taught that we can train the brain to think about how to fix things instead of focusing on what's broken.

As a result, I oriented myself to be "solution-focused" rather than "problem-solving." This is the kind of language that I use with kids in my practice: "Okay, that's the problem, now let's think about some solutions."

Thought Replacements

This is a really great tool for teaching a kid who may have low self-esteem or generally tends to assume the worst. These kinds of kids have what I call "a little birdie" in their heads telling them "Nobody wants to play with me!" or "I'm bad at pitching in baseball!" Or "I'm bad at math!"

Of course, as a parent, when your child says these things aloud to you, your first instinct will be to act as your child's cheerleader and contradict him: "Of course people want to play with you!" "Of course, you're good at pitching!" "Of course, you're good at math!" But if you only contradict your child, you're just sending him the message that he's gotten it wrong. When you offer your child a "thought replacement" instead of a contradiction, you're validating how he feels while giving him a way to reframe the situation.

When he says, "I'm bad at math!" you can say, "Hmmm . . . You know, instead of saying you're bad at math, could you just say math is hard for you? The way I see it, you put a lot of extra effort into math because you find it difficult. Maybe you could say that you just have to work extra hard at math? What do you think?"

In this scenario, you're not telling your child that he's going to be a math superstar, and you're not telling him to stop feeling the way he's feeling, but you're emphasizing his effort (which gives him room to change and grow) rather than his belief that he's innately bad at something.

This kind of thought replacement or reframing can be a really powerful tool to teach a child to do for himself. If a child feels bad about something and he doesn't learn to think about it differently, then he can get stuck in a negative feedback loop: he believes he's bad at math so therefore he ends up being bad at math. This is what we call a self-fulfilling prophecy: repeated thoughts that are assigned proof or evidence become beliefs, and our beliefs can convert to our reality, especially at this young age. *Reframing* pushes a child to consider that growth and change are possible for him. I tell the kids I work with, "You know, you can change what the little birdie is telling you. But if you don't work on changing it, it will keep telling you that you're bad at something, and we don't want that to happen."

"The Volcano," "The Iceberg," and "The Tornado"

Many parents and children in my practice find it helpful when we use easy-to-understand images to talk about and process feelings and emotions. Emotions can seem so amorphous and intangible that visual metaphors can really help. I'll often draw these three images on the whiteboard in my office so we can all refer back to them. You may find it helpful to introduce these images to your child as well.

THE VOLCANO

This is the image I use when a child is struggling with anger and is prone to outbursts: something triggers the child, the lava starts bubbling, then the volcano explodes. Giving parents and kids a shared language around what happens before, during, and after the volcano erupts can be really helpful. *Before* a volcano explodes, the lava is bubbling on the inside. If you see your kid is starting to get angry you could say, "Hey, what's bubbling in there?," which is a slightly lighter, less intimidating way of saying, "What's wrong?" If your child erupts at everyone in the family, *during* this outburst you can say, "I know that yesterday things were bubbling at school. Seems like you got home, and the bubbling became a big eruption. Hot lava is flowing everywhere right now!" *After* the event, you can use this same language to discuss what happened. "So what happened when the lava spilled down? We ended up with a big mess and a lot of people got hurt. Now we have to clean up that lava before it hardens. And even if it does harden, we can still move the molten rocks."

Remember that we're not trying to deny or get rid of the anger. Anger can be a healthy emotion—it's a part of normal self-expression and communication. You don't want to send your child the message that they are never going to erupt—you want them to know that anger is an intense feeling that can be healthy to let out when it's still bubbling before he gets to the point of explosion when he no longer feels in control. You can tell your child: "Anger is normal. It will come and go. I want you to be able to understand why you are feeling like this and then express it in a constructive way. I want you to feel in control, not like an eruption where we end up with a big mess and a lot to clean up."

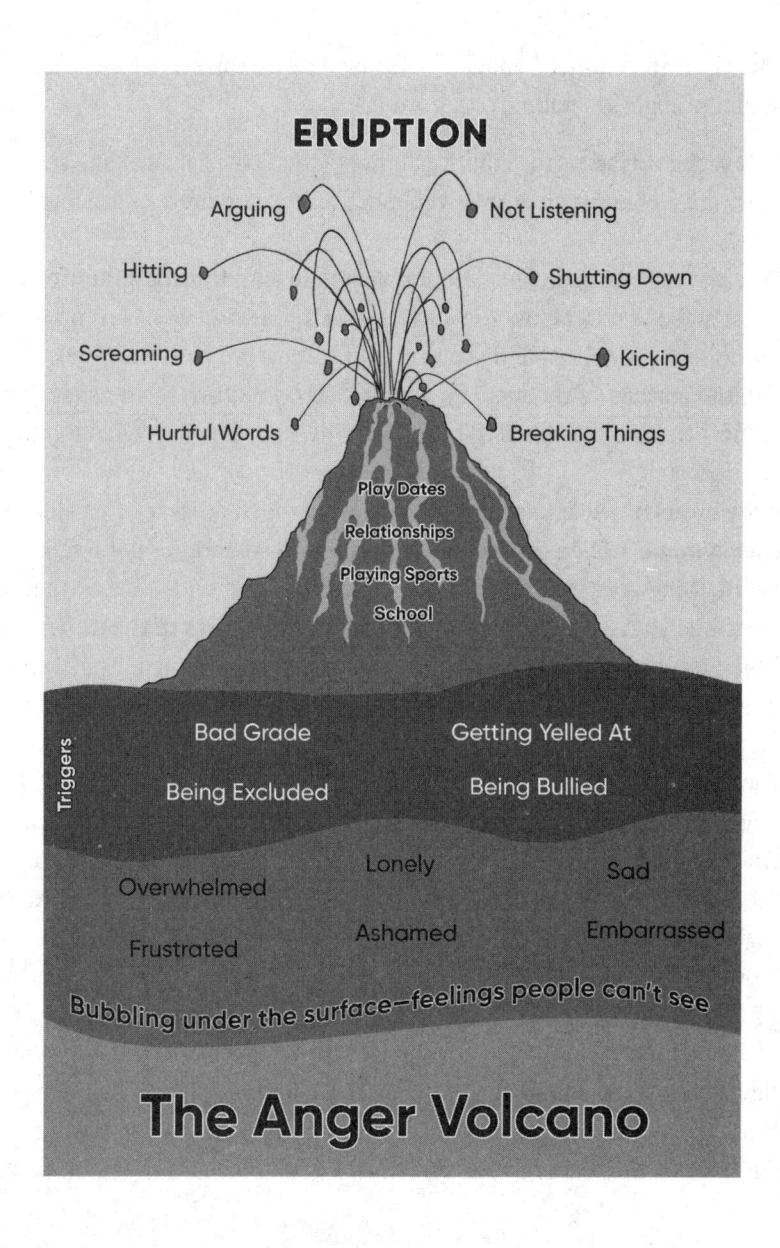

ERUPTION

- Arguing
- Not Listening
- Hitting
- Shutting Down
- Screaming
- Kicking
- Hurtful Words
- Breaking Things

Play Dates
Relationships
Playing Sports
School

Triggers

Bad Grade
Getting Yelled At
Being Excluded
Being Bullied

Overwhelmed
Lonely
Sad
Frustrated
Ashamed
Embarrassed

Bubbling under the surface—feelings people can't see

The Anger Volcano

THE ICEBERG

This is an image I use with parents and children to help explain that a child's behavior is only the tip of the iceberg and that there are usually some pretty deep emotions hiding below the surface we can't see. When I describe this to families, I split the iceberg into two parts:

The tip is the surface behavior—this is what we can see—for example smiling, laughing, yelling, or ignoring.

Below the surface is the emotional state—this is the part we can't see—these are feelings such as overwhelmed, guilty, pressured, or ashamed.

You can talk through the iceberg with your child, helping him to identify what's above and below the surface. Let's imagine your eleven-year-old comes home from school and snaps moodily at everyone in the house. If you stay on the surface of the iceberg, you would say, "Why are you snapping at everyone?" Instead, you need to begin your investigation into what's going on below the water.

Start by acknowledging the tip: "You've snapped at each of us since you have been home." Then go deeper: "I notice you sometimes get cranky with us if something goes wrong at school." If you are met with silence, then you can continue your investigation into the less visible parts of the iceberg. Is it possible he's forgotten his homework, misplaced something, or he's worried about a bully at school? Could he have had a fight with his best friend, fallen during basketball practice, or given a wrong answer in class and been laughed at? You can say, "I know that you had basketball today. How did it go?" Or "I know you've been feeling pretty stressed about the test that's coming up."

Once again, you don't need to figure everything out the second your child gets home. If he is staying pretty quiet, you can say, "I can tell you don't want to talk right now and that's okay, I'm going to make your snack." Letting him know that you understand, but that you're going to proceed, will lessen the tension far more than if you continue with an interrogation. Sometimes, if you let things go in the moment, what's beneath the iceberg will reveal itself later, often at bedtime, when you are holding emotional space for him without distraction.

If it seems like your child does want to engage with you, you can always remind him of the iceberg. You can draw out the iceberg together, naming the tip and the bottom and filling in what's going on under there. It may take some time for a child to understand what's happening below the surface of his behaviors, but with practice, thinking about his emotions and behavior in this way will help him gain both greater self-awareness and also the ability to see things from other people's perspective.

When Ryan's mom, Jaime, learned about the iceberg she told me, "Now I feel like I have something to do when Ryan is in a mood! I have a job to do. I have to figure out what's going on under that mood. Before, I'd just see Ryan talking back to me and it made me want to yell at him to stop! Now, I can ask myself, 'What's under the surface?'"

THE TORNADO

This is an image that I use with children who are having a hard time "decentering." Decentering is when you step back from your immediate thoughts, feelings, and experiences and observe them from a more objective and detached perspective, shifting your focus from a narrow view to a broader awareness of what's going on. It's a concept I use from the acceptance and commitment therapy (ACT) framework.

When I'm talking about decentering with families, I'll draw a spiraling tornado on my whiteboard. Then I explain that when a child's really upset it's like he's at the bottom of the tornado, where things are most concentrated, and where the damage gets done. But if he can wind his way out of the tornado toward the top, he can begin to see the bigger picture. In fact, things keep getting calmer and calmer as he winds upward, until he's flying above the tornado and can see the whole view.

At this point, that child will usually ask how he can wind his way up? I prompt him to imagine floating up to the top. In order to float up, he needs to calm his body, let go of what he's holding on to, and just observe. The goal is to detach from whatever is happening on the ground, even if for just a few seconds, to get a better look from up above.

For example, your child may get into an argument with his sister, who didn't want to share a toy. He may get fixated on the fact she won't share, lashing out at her, making her cry, and then telling you, "It's her fault, she hates me, and she doesn't want to play with me!" At this point, your child is at the bottom of the tornado, where it's intense and damaging. But if you can remind him to wind his way up through the tornado by releasing the thought that she hates him, this frees up mental space to remember that his sister only just got the toy. He can then rethink the situation: "She just got it, it's a new toy, she doesn't want to share it with anyone right now." In this situation, you can remind your child about the image of the tornado or even draw it out, naming the different parts and filling them in together.

Stop, Breathe, Think, *Then* Act

One of my favorite homemade tools to use when I'm working on self-regulation with kids is Stop, Breathe, Think, *Then* Act, or "Stop and Think" for short. This is a strategy your child can practice whenever he's experiencing big emotions, so he can respond appropriately, rather than lashing out or shutting down. Here's how it works: your child comes up against something that triggers him. Let's say he comes home, and his little brother has destroyed the LEGO car in his bedroom. He starts heading down the hall to his brother's room while warning that he is going to destroy something of his. In this case, there isn't a lot of time to act. You need a tool that is understood by you and your child and can be used right away:

1. The first step is to STOP. When I say stop, I truly mean your child should freeze in place, slam on the brakes.
2. Then he needs to BREATHE, in and out, deep breaths, three to five times.
3. Once he has done his breathing (which should take about thirty seconds), he can THINK: "I am so angry right now, what should I do? What will happen if I walk into my brother's room?"
4. Your child needs to do all of these steps before he ACTS, like deciding to go to the kitchen to tell his babysitter what happened.

"Stop and Think" is something your child can practice and then ideally do for himself. It's intended to be self-guided; he does not need to be told to do it. Even so, a prompt is helpful as a reminder once he's learned this technique. In my office I keep a stop sign that I can point to when we're practicing. You can have the same sign at home or signal to your child "time-out" with your hands, prompting him to begin the "Stop and Think" technique because you can see he really needs it. By practicing "Stop and Think," over time, this language will become the voice in your child's head, guiding him toward controlling impulsive behavior.

"Stop and Think" is a great tool for adults, as well. So, if you find yourself using it and it's working, mention it to your child. The more you can model how to manage your anger and control your big feelings, the better he will be able to incorporate these strategies into his daily life.

The Importance of Giving Your Child Some Control

Many times, kids will tell me that when they experience big, intense feelings, it seems to them as if they are not in control of themselves, as if someone else is controlling what they say and do. Although it may sound counterintuitive, one of the best ways to help an out-of-control child calm down is to help him to focus on something he can control.

Imagine your child is having a meltdown because he doesn't want to pack up his clothes for a trip to visit his grandparents. As a parent, it may seem as if you have a couple of options here: you can simply demand that your child pack up his clothes and threaten to punish him if he doesn't, or you can do the packing for him. If you demand your child pack his clothes and threaten to punish him, he's likely to continue melting down (remember he feels totally out of control right now, and you're taking even more control away from him by threatening to punish him). If you pack his things for him, you're sending him the message that he's incapable of packing up his things. Kids whose parents do things for them because it's "easier" can develop more problems in the long run as this disempowers children and can actually negatively impact their self-esteem. Here's a third approach. Instead of demanding he pack or doing it for him, you can say to your child, "I'll help you pack. Do you want to do the underwear or the shirts first?" By asking your child this question, you're getting him to focus on something he can control, while still getting the outcome you want, which is that he packs up his things so

> you can leave. Get him started on the task, send him the message that he can handle this—and your child is much more likely to comply.

Mindfulness Techniques

Mindfulness is key for both self-awareness and self-regulation in kids. Studies show that over time, practicing mindfulness techniques such as breathing and meditation actually thickens the cerebral cortex, including the prefrontal cortex, which is responsible for perception and reasoning. It reduces activity in the amygdala, which governs the brain's fight-or-flight impulse. Researchers from MIT have found that students who received mindfulness training in middle school showed better academic performance, received fewer suspensions, and reported less stress than those who did not receive the training.[2]

Mindfulness also allows for better social connections, friendships, and relationships. It can help with attention regulation—deciding what you're going to focus on. Mindfulness can give a child greater control over cognitive distortions or faulty and inaccurate beliefs. These distortions include polarized thinking (school is always good or always bad) or overgeneralization (big dogs bite people). By practicing mindfulness, the child learns to change what the voice in his head is telling him.

Early in my career I trained as a children's yoga instructor because I wanted to learn more about how movement and breath work affects kids and how to teach them to use these skills. Here are some of my favorite mindfulness training exercises specifically for kids ages six to twelve, including breath work, progressive muscle relaxation, and mindful movement, such as yoga. Even just a few minutes of mindfulness a day, most days a week, can have a noticeable impact on attention, mood, and quality of relationships.

BREATHING

Paying attention to your breath is one of the most effective ways to calm the central nervous system. When you focus on your breathing, you slow down, and can look inward instead of outward (which is what you often see in dys-

The Unexpected Emotional Ups and Downs of Middle Childhood   133

regulation). Breath awareness involves paying attention to the depth, rhythm, and quality of breath. All of this can have a profound impact on relaxation and stress management.

Here are some simple breathing techniques:

- Belly breathing. You can start by teaching your child to place one hand on his belly and one hand on his chest so he can feel the rise and fall of his breath and begin to center himself.
- Box breathing. This can be a great technique to teach your child as a starting point. It's a four-count exercise that can be done anywhere. Have your child take a deep, slow breath in while counting to four. Now hold that breath for another count of four. Then slowly exhale, also on a count of four. And finally, hold that exhale for a final count of four. And repeat. It's called "box breathing" because you can imagine going around a square on your counts of four.
- The four, seven, eight breathing technique. This involves breathing in for four seconds, holding the breath for seven seconds, and exhaling for eight seconds. You can also have your child breathe in for four seconds as he scrunches up his face; hold the position tightly for seven seconds, then breathe out. Repeat for the shoulders, hands, down to the toes.
- Another approach I've found helpful especially for young children is to use images to describe a certain type of breath. A "flower breath" is when you imagine your chest opening up like a flower when you inhale. A "candle breath" is when you imagine blowing a candle out as you exhale. A "bumblebee breath" is when you make a *bzzzzz* noise as you exhale and a "snake breath" is when you make a *ssssss* noise. "Breathing buddies" is when you breathe in sync with one another.

NATURE IMMERSION

You don't need to be in a forest or even a park to do this easy mindfulness exercise. You can simply step outside with your child, even onto a sidewalk. Then you purposefully look and listen for the sounds and sights of nature. Set an intention. Can you spot five clouds? Hear two birds singing? Find six different kinds of leaves? Find a feather or dandelion weed to blow? Describe the color of the sky as precisely as possible. This exercise helps stop racing thoughts and rumination and gets kids out of their heads and into a calmer frame of mind and body.

MANTRAS AND POSITIVE AFFIRMATIONS

This is a technique that doesn't work for everyone. For example, Ryan has never taken to it. But I do have a patient named Avery who loves to do mantras and positive affirmations. She has a lot of avoidance because of anxiety—and so she uses her mantras to help her overcome that. She says to herself, "I am brave and strong" over and over until she believes it, at least in that moment. She writes sticky notes that say "I am brave and strong, I can do this, I've done this before," and she puts them around her room, in her school folders, and on the bathroom mirror. When a child repeats mantras or positive affirmations, it begins to rewire the brain. If you say something enough, if you hear it enough, your brain will no longer reject the message.

YOGA, MEDITATION, AND MOVEMENT

Yoga is a practice that has been around for five thousand years for a reason: it really works. Research shows that yoga can be extremely helpful with stress management and overall mental health, reducing anxiety and depression, and helping the brain to function better. Practicing yoga strengthens parts of the brain that play a key role in memory, attention, awareness, thought, and language, and may improve executive functioning, something that kids of this age are still developing. Brain imaging indicates that people who regularly practice yoga have a thicker cerebral cortex (the area of the brain responsible for information processing) and hippocampus (the area of the brain involved in learning and memory) compared with those who don't. Not only is yoga good for cognitive functioning, doing yoga poses can boost your child's mood by lowering levels of stress hormones, increasing the production of feel-good neurotransmitters known as endorphins, and bringing more oxygenated blood to the brain. And according to a Harvard Health review, it can uniquely improve a person's mood by elevating levels of a brain chemical called gamma-aminobutyric acid (GABA), which is associated with improved mood and decreased anxiety.[3]

My favorite yoga tool for kids is the Yoga Pretzels card deck, which has fifty cards illustrated with yoga poses and breathing techniques and is available online. Each card describes a different pose or technique that you can easily replicate with your child. There are also many free YouTube videos you can access and follow.

Meditation is another great practice to teach your child. Regular meditation has been shown to decrease amygdala activity, the part of the brain dedicated to emotional processing, which helps to regulate the stress response. As emotional reactivity decreases, your child may have a more even-keeled response when faced with a problem or stressful event. To encourage your child to meditate, you can begin by choosing a calm and quiet environment like a bedroom that is hopefully also a comfortable space for your child to sit, eyes closed, in one position for a few minutes. Reducing distractions will help create an environment ideal for being still and present. Then ask your child to focus on an image or a thought and see if he can hold it in his mind. You could read a guided meditation out loud to him (these are available online, in books available at the library and in app stores). You could use prompts such as asking him to imagine lying in the grass or floating in water. You can even have him listen to apps or videos that can vary in length and age appropriateness. Before you know it, your child will have drifted off to a calmer and more relaxing place. If you can, meditate alongside him, so you are both in that state of calm together. Start with short sessions so that your child doesn't get bored or tired but can feel successful, as if maybe he could have gone on longer. With practice you can increase the time you spend meditating together as your child gets interested or motivated by the challenge of it, eventually doing it on his own.

But you aren't limited to meditation or yoga to practice mindfulness. Other simple physical activities such as dancing, going for a walk, running, or even just stretching can have a mindfulness effect when done with intention. When your child does this, he is training his brain to focus, which has lasting effects even when under stress.

Body Awareness

Body awareness is the conscious perception and understanding of your own body and its various sensations, movements, and positions in space. It involves being attuned to the physical aspects of your body, including sensations, emotions, and physiological responses. Body awareness plays a crucial role in overall well-being, self-regulation, and the mind-body connection. Since emotions manifest physically in the body, awareness of what's going on inside includes recognizing and understanding the physical sensations associated with different emotions, such as stress leading to muscle tension in your shoulders or worries leading to butterflies in the stomach. It can be especially helpful to teach your child to recognize tension or discomfort in his body, and to address those issues through relaxation techniques such as breathing, stretching, or other kinds of self-care. One useful technique to teach your child is to do a "body scan," which enables a kid to slow down to better understand his body and its connection to mental and emotional states and the behaviors that follow.

Here's how to do a body scan:

Your child can sit, lie down, or stand up. You can tell him, "That situation happened when you got really upset. Let's go through what was taking place in every part of your body and the five senses while that was happening. What were you seeing? What were you hearing? What were you smelling? Did your mouth feel dry? Were you clenching your jaw? Did your shoulders and neck tense up? Was your heart racing? Did you have a stomachache? What about your hands? And your feet?" And go all the way down through your child's body to his toes. Remember, you're just getting your child to report these sensations to you; you're not making any judgments or correcting him in any way—it's just about recognizing what's happening in the body.

Then you can let your child know that clenching fists, grinding teeth, curling toes, hunching shoulders, and tensing our bodies in general are all ways that the body stores stress and if he becomes aware of that, he can move in ways that let that stress go. He can get up and stretch. He can run around the room. He can punch a pillow. He can do a goofy dance or, like Taylor Swift says, he can shake it off.

Another component of body awareness is how you use your body language to communicate with others. Body language can include the way we move, our postures, and gestures. I often point out to kids that their posture tells a story and I can tell how they are feeling by looking at how their shoulders are slumped, or how they are walking, or how they are building with blocks. I'll say, "I notice every time you talk about your math teacher your head goes down or your leg starts shaking or you start fidgeting. What do you think your body is telling you?" If I can teach a child that his body is a vessel of emotional information, then I'm also teaching him to trust his gut, an invaluable life skill. If you can set your child up to understand his body, he can be more in touch with his "gut" or intuition as an older teen and young adult.

You can also flip this kind of awareness for your child, explaining to him that he can use his body to make himself feel more confident and less nervous. "Could your body pretend you feel really good about your presentation in front of the class next week? Stand with your shoulders back, chin up, feet apart." Even if the child doesn't start out feeling confident, that feeling will grow in him as he assumes a confident stance.

Looking Ahead

In the not-so-distant future your child will be a teenager and may find himself the target of pressures either in person or online that you likely won't know anything about. By practicing self-regulation and mindfulness with your child now, these skills will become second nature, serving him well when he needs to "Stop and Think" about what to do in new situations, helping him slow down long enough so that he doesn't react impulsively, possibly getting himself into trouble by trying to defend himself or someone else.

In a Nutshell

When your child learns to self-regulate using some or any of the techniques above, he'll begin thinking before he acts. He'll come up with alternative approaches and solutions to challenges. He'll be in better control of his outbursts, holding back on crying and whining and learning to calm himself. He'll know when and where big feelings can safely be expressed. He'll handle disappointments through talking about feelings and work through his fears using coping skills. He'll ask for help instead of getting highly frustrated. He'll use empathy to a greater degree and learn to reframe problems, putting them into context and perspective. He'll find it easier to transition from one activity to another and to work cooperatively in groups. And your attempts to set boundaries will be met with a much greater success rate as a result.

You can teach your child to better self-regulate by:

- Helping him become a feelings detective
- Giving him a wide range of words to describe his feelings and emotions so he can correctly identify them
- Guiding him to identify his triggers, proactively plan around them, and come up with alternative solutions
- Helping him with thought replacements
- Teaching him about the volcano, the iceberg and the tornado
- Showing him how to do the "Stop and Think" technique
- Giving him some control when he feels out of control
- Teaching him mindfulness techniques such as yoga, meditation, and breathing
- Introducing him to body awareness

In time and with practice, your child will absorb these skills and no longer need you to prompt him to do them, giving him a foundation for how to move through life's challenges, attuned to his own feelings and emotions, and able to talk about them with you and with himself in ways that are productive and not destructive. In the coming chapters, we're going to look at the many kinds of issues you're going to face now that your child is in middle childhood. With your child's emotional foundation (and yours) in place, you're going to find that these sometimes challenging situations and conversations will become a whole lot easier to approach.

CHAPTER 5

Pressure

School, Social, Sports

Challenging behavior occurs when the demands and expectations being placed upon a child outstrip the skills they have to respond.

—Dr. Ross Greene

Cici was in eighth grade when she first came to see me. Even though she was only thirteen years old, she was already suffering from chronic exhaustion and anxiety. As I quickly learned, the root causes of her difficulties went all the way back to elementary school. Cici told me that even in fourth and fifth grade, she'd felt the pressure to succeed at school. The night before her fifth-grade exams she couldn't stop making flash cards and reviewing them, unable to fall asleep until they were all memorized. Then she would wake up extra early to review her notes again. As Cici recalled, when her parents noticed she was up early, they praised her, telling her they were sure no one else was up at 5:30 a.m. studying.

When I shared with Cici's parents that their daughter's symptoms of anxiety and self-reported levels of stress were high—and dated back to elementary school—they were confused. They told me her grades had always been excellent, and while they did see her working hard, they also felt that she was naturally bright and high achieving. "Well, something has to set her apart, we do expect a lot out of her," they explained to me. Now that Cici was in eighth grade, and private high school applications and interviews were in progress—with that being the main topic anyone talked about—what Cici's parents didn't see coming was that she was burning out. Not only was she playing on a travel field hockey team, but she was also missing homework deadlines and procrastinating about completing her applications for high school. She couldn't keep up the pace.

Cici was conflicted and at times said things like she didn't care and she wasn't going to try anymore. Cici was struggling with what we call the perfectionism-procrastination loop. In our sessions together, we worked on having a better understanding of what this meant for her. Perfectionism and procrastination can start to loop where perfectionism and fear of failure (or what I call fear of not getting it right the very first time) causes procrastination (or what I also call avoidance), which can lead to increased anxiety and stress. Cici initially didn't understand what I was talking about or what was happening, but her fear of failure on top of chronic exhaustion from trying to be the best at everything was causing her to avoid important deadlines, including her capstone project, and to no longer feel confident enough to speak in front of the class.

It took a couple of months to shift the expectations bar for Cici. It wasn't that the bar got so low that she wasn't doing her schoolwork, but, as I explained to Cici and her parents, it couldn't be as high as the one she'd set for herself in the past or she was going to burn out completely. Cici was initially hesitant to do this work because she feared letting go of this impossibly high bar—which she felt was important to her identity. Her parents were also cautious. They were concerned that Cici would stop performing at a high enough level, and if this happened, they felt it would diminish her prospects for college, feeding into Cici's perfectionism.

Parents often have a tough time acknowledging this, but real damage is caused when we put too much pressure on our children to succeed. The term "parental pressure" is real. This has been studied extensively, and although much of the data points to what happens to children when they are pressured, it generally shows up as depression, anxiety, self-harm, and eating disorders. According to the APA, perfectionism is the tendency to demand of others or of oneself an extremely high or even flawless level of performance, in excess of what is required by the situation, and is associated with depression, anxiety, eating disorders, and other mental health problems. Parental pressure and perfectionism have very similar outcomes. Kids are rewarded by parents, coaches, and teachers for setting an extremely high bar for themselves and working tirelessly to attain their goals, even at the expense of their friendships, downtime, socializing, even just the freedom to do nothing. The expectations that parents set for children are well-intended—wanting your kid to do well, maybe better than you did—but can easily create an unhealthy mindset in a child like Cici, who thought she always needed to be the best, the smartest, the fastest, and most talented in the room, or she had no self-worth.

The qualities of perfectionism (studying above and beyond, writing an essay over and over, only doing things that you are really good at) that lead to praise and recognition in the elementary and middle school years too often lead to burnout in high school. I have a lot of experience with this. I often say that I could rename my therapy center the Anxiety Center, and this isn't because nearly 10 percent of US children have a diagnosed anxiety disorder; it's because I happen to see a significant amount of highly gifted and talented (HGT) kids and teens in my practice. These kids aren't just particularly bright, they are also very anxious, and they tend to put a high degree of pressure on themselves. An Arizona State University study of 506 sixth graders showed the ways this kind of pressure can often backfire. The students were asked to rank the top values of their parents: three values related to achievement and three related to kindness toward others. Researchers found that the students who believed their parents valued achievement more than kindness *actually did worse academically and socially*.

Perfectionism can become a lifelong trait, and research has shown that perfectionists become more neurotic and less conscientious as they get older. Perfectionism is also a trait that appears to get handed down in families, with perfectionist parents raising perfectionist children. A 2022 meta-analysis of existing research on perfectionism found that parental expectations may be more damaging than parental criticism in this respect. "Young people internalize those expectations and depend on them for their self-esteem," the APA published research stated. "And when they fail to meet them, as they invariably will, they'll be critical of themselves for not matching up. To compensate, they strive to be perfect."

This kind of pressure to be perfect starts as early as preschool and continues through the elementary years and into middle and high school. In the process, parents overschedule their kids, hire tutors to help them secure good grades, lose appreciation for carefree time in childhood, and engage in the engineering of their social lives. Meanwhile, most of these parents can look back on their own childhoods with memories of plenty of unscheduled time to run around outside, staying out until dark unsupervised, or playing rudimentary video games. The problem is, they aren't granting their kids the same freedoms. The increasing cost and competition to get coveted college spots and scholarships is panicking adults, who are forcing their children into more academic, athletic, and extracurricular pursuits. Compared to the late 1980s, kids' perceptions of their parents' expectations have increased about 40 percent. In their efforts to shape a "well-rounded" child, however, parents are proving to be clumsy sculptors, resulting in unstable children who are so busy they don't have time to play or, frankly, to learn life skills. This is partly why so many of them wind up in my office.

So here's a little dose of tough love for parents of all backgrounds who feel the need to pressure children to succeed: your primary concern should be on raising mentally, physically, and emotionally healthy children, rather than successful applicants. Instead of focusing on grooming your child for a competitive high school spot or enrolling her in seven days a week of activities, sports, and tutoring to build up a résumé by age seventeen, you can help her manage pressure from within—or from outside—by teaching her that failure is normal, natural, and necessary. Focus on her *efforts*, not test scores, and this will help her to develop a healthy sense of self and curiosity, which we know is correlated to better achievement and mental health outcomes. If you are reading this knowing that you lie somewhere on the perfectionism continuum yourself, be aware that you may be passing these traits on to your child and adjust accordingly.

After a few months of working together, Cici was able to find a better balance by creating boundaries for homework (one and a half hours a night), sports (ninety minutes, six days a week), and doing nothing (thirty minutes a night). Cici and I also made a deal that she was only allowed to ask for reassurance once from her parents (versus repeatedly asking them if they were sure what she did/wrote was good enough) and then one round of editing for herself after finishing work, along with one homework pass a month (which the school allowed students to earn but she never cashed in). We also worked on her excessive list making and organizational systems. We decided that she would have one master list for the week that had subcategories instead of different lists that she would write and rewrite several times a week, often containing things to do that were far in advance.

Over time, Cici's parents realized the pressure they were putting on their daughter was counterproductive. Once they saw that her anxiety was beginning to cause her to shut down, and that she was going to practice healthier versions of what she had already been doing, they understood this was the right approach. Soon enough, they saw their child starting to relax, smile more, and be less irritable. Cici found her balance, and while she is still a high-achieving student athlete, she no longer has such extreme anxiety and routines that were exhausting her. She's even tried new things like performing in a school musical, and even though she wasn't by her own standards "the best," she said she was "good enough" and had fun! This was a big goal that she worked hard on—being good enough and allowing herself to have fun—and one that I know she took with her as she transitioned into high school.

> **PARADIGM SHIFT**
>
> **Paradigm:** My child is growing up in an extremely competitive world. I need to do everything in my power to ensure a successful future for him. Even at this young age, I need to make sure he is advanced at school and in sports as well as enrolled in multiple activities if he wants to be successful someday.
>
> **Shift:** Parents need to reprioritize their values to place a child's mental health and well-being ahead of their ambitions for academic or athletic success, even if that means reducing how many activities children can participate in and how much time they spend studying.

How to Help Your Child Succeed at School *Without* Applying Pressure

Many parents I meet with tell me they feel like they're being a bad parent if they *don't* put pressure on children to succeed. They feel as if they would be "giving up" or failing to help that child to "fulfill his true potential." These parents are either overachievers themselves or perhaps feel as if their parents didn't push them hard enough or see other parents pushing their kids and fear their own child is "falling behind." These parents care deeply about their kids and want them to succeed. So, when I tell them parental pressure can actually backfire and be detrimental to kids, they often tell me they no longer know how to be good parents.

In fact, there are many ways that you can help your child to succeed *without* applying pressure. Number one is to allow your child more autonomy so he can develop a sense of mastery. When you send your child the message that he's capable of doing his own laundry or going to the corner store alone to pick up an ingredient for dinner, or taking care of a pet without your help, this will encourage him to become competent in other areas of his life as well. Make sure you give your child enough space to try new things on his own, rather than always leaping to help him. Let him fail at these tasks sometimes. When you do this, you give him the opportunity to course correct—and this will increase his sense of his innate capabilities.

Remember it's only fairly recently that parents have felt it necessary to hover over young children, supervising their every move. A 1946 advice column in *Parents* magazine described the case of a child "not yet two years old" who liked playing in the yard when her mother was with her but would cry and want to be taken inside if mom went inside to do her work. The mother figured out that the child cried not from fear of being alone outdoors, but from fear that she could not get into the house by herself if she wanted to. The problem was solved by lowering the door latch so the child could open and close the door herself. The result, according to the author, was that "now she plays happily in the yard for hours, on good days."

A 1956 article in *Parents* expressed approval of a mother's decision to acquiesce to her five-year-old's desire to walk to school by himself, about four blocks from home. The article made it clear that if a child is old enough for kindergarten, then that child is old enough to find his or her own way to and from school without an adult.

A 1966 article in *Good Housekeeping* proposed a set of guidelines for children's autonomy as follows: "A six- to eight-year-old can be expected to follow simple routes to school, be able to find a telephone or report to a policeman if he is lost, and to know he must call home if he is going to be late. A nine- to eleven-year-old should be able to travel on public buses and streetcars, apply some simple first aid, and exercise reasonable judgment in many unfamiliar situations." Compare these expectations with a 2006 article in *Good Housekeeping* titled, "Are You a Good Mother?" The article made it clear that the answer is yes only if you closely watch and supervise your child pretty much all of the time.

If your child is scheduled so tightly and has so much homework he doesn't have time for tasks around the house such as feeding a pet or picking up his things—and if you never allow him to participate in simple chores and make mistakes while doing them—then you need to switch your priorities. Think about the ways that children were empowered in the past at much younger ages and find ways to foster that sense of independence in your child. That doesn't mean that your six-year-old should necessarily start walking to school alone, but it does mean that you could set the expectation that he cleans up his room and put away his own things. By giving your child chores around the house, this will enrich your child's sense of competency, which will lead to greater confidence in other areas too.

Here are some other tips for helping your child to succeed without applying pressure:

- Make time for free play. When a child aged six to twelve has time to play, he has the opportunity to use his imagination, make mistakes, be creative, and let off steam, along with many other benefits. This is one of the most important things you can do to help your child grow up to be a healthy, happy high schooler *and* college student.
- Praise your child sparingly and specifically. The amount of praise I hear in my office and wider community gives me pause. Parents today tell their kids they do a "good job" when they do anything: get out of the car, strike out, walk into school, say hello to a stranger. When you praise indiscriminately, it becomes meaningless to a child. Instead of praising every little thing, praise when you see your child applying *effort*. Even if your child gets an A, don't praise the grade, praise the hard work that went into the grade.
- Model and help your child develop emotional intelligence or the ability to identify, understand, and manage one's own emotions and the emotions of others. Talk about emotions with your child, help him to identify when he is feeling a certain way and how to channel that feeling appropriately— and do the same for yourself.

- Give your child age-appropriate opportunities to earn money. Whether it's having a lemonade stand or helping out with yard work, finding ways for your child to earn money can reinforce a sense of creativity and achievement.
- Develop and maintain systems that work for your child to help him learn organization and studying skills. Feeling organized can increase feelings of competency and decrease stress. Middle school is an especially critical time to focus on these skills because this is usually when we ask more of students than their still-developing brains can manage.
- Value kindness in your child. Explain to him that the most important thing he can do is to be a kind friend, family member, and community member. When you set this expectation for your child, studies show that it will actually help him in all aspects of his life.

The Race-to-College Mindset and How to Avoid It

Somewhere between our college application days and the present day, the admissions process has morphed into a race to turn children into super-teens that have stacked résumés, letters of recommendation from senators, world travels, state championship trophies, speech and debate medals, and service hours in developing countries. Parents are plagued with anxiety that their child needs above A grades (have you noticed how many kids have a 4.5+ GPA?), near-perfect scores on the SAT, and a list of colleges twenty-five deep that they are going to spend two years traveling to half of them to check off the box that says they toured in person.

As a result, many well-resourced parents are sending their kids to summer enrichment programs starting at ages eleven and twelve (yes, you read that right) at prestigious universities like Oxford University in the UK. Yale University offers "a rigorous six-week summer program for *highly motivated middle schoolers* looking to challenge themselves academically. The goal of the program is to help students get a head start by equipping them with the academic skills necessary for them to excel *in college*" (italics added). This program (and others) accepts *rising* sixth graders—a rising sixth grader can be just ten years old! The summer before sixth grade they are still losing baby teeth, they still need lots of play and physical activity to help them develop, and they are still in the middle of significant cognitive development. They are learning to think more abstractly, but their reasoning skills and ability to grasp complex concepts are under construction. Most children at this age *do not* need to be sent off to a summer program at a prestigious university but rather would benefit from playing with friends or going to good old-fashioned summer camp and maybe an enrichment program that can stimulate their minds during the summer months.

As a parent, you have a choice. You can follow others down the path of panicking about your child's future, or you can decide to have a different mindset. When you prioritize your young child's mental health over his academic success, you are setting him on a path for a happier and better-adjusted life—with the added benefit that he will be more likely to cope with the demands of high school once he gets there.

Social Pressure in School: Bullying

In third grade for girls and fourth grade for boys, we see shifting social dynamics at school paired with increased demands in academics and homework. Navigating friendships and fitting in become even more important in a child's life, with social dynamics often becoming a source of stress and conflict. Prior to these grades, when your child felt left out on the playground, you could easily say things like "Well, maybe tomorrow will be a good day to play with other friends" or "It's okay for Josie to want to play with another friend sometimes, I bet tomorrow the three of you will play." But now, helping your child navigate social stress becomes more complicated, and with puberty starting earlier in many kids, these changes often show up at the emotional level.

Sadly, bullying can begin in preschool and kindergarten, and it peaks in middle school. By bullying, I mean the textbook definition, which is the repetitive, intentional hurting of one person or group by another person or group, where the relationship involves an imbalance of power. These three elements must exist for it to be considered bullying—it must be repetitive, intentional, and involve a power differential. In my practice, many kids use the term "being bullied" fairly often to describe how they are being treated by someone else. I make sure that I help them to distinguish true bullying from kids just being mean. There is a difference. Bullying is meant to threaten, harm, and intimidate another person. It is about power and control. Being mean is disregarding someone's feelings and it certainly works—it is hurtful, but the intention is different.

There are six different types of bullying: physical, verbal, relational, cyber-, sexual, and prejudicial bullying.

- **Physical** bullying is the most obvious type as it involves physical aggression, making it easier to spot.
- **Verbal** bullying is harder to discern for adults, and kids can deny or downplay insults and intimidation, yet this is the most common form of bullying and the type that is likely to go on the longest and causes great stress and anxiety.
- **Relational** bullying (aka relational aggression) involves actions intended to harm someone's reputation or relationships by embarrassing him around others, spreading rumors, purposely leaving him out of social situations, or ostracizing him from a group. As school-age children become more aware of social dynamics, they use these dynamics to manipulate social hierarchies to get what they want. And while relational aggression is carried out more by girls than it is with boys, certainly both boys and girls can threaten, hurt, or intimidate others using any and all forms of bullying.
- **Cyberbullying** happens online through phones and tablets using texting or social media apps and involves posting or sending harmful content, including messages and photos that typically result in humiliation, shame, and violation through rapid sharing and reposts. We see this peak in middle school as more kids get smart phones and social media accounts.
- **Sexual** bullying involves using sexual comments, gestures, or actions to hurt, embarrass, or intimidate someone. This type of bullying is more likely to occur in middle and high school.
- **Prejudicial** (aka racial) bullying involves online or in-person bullying based on someone's race, ethnicity, religion, or sexual orientation. This type of bullying is based on stereotypes and is often a result of the belief that some people deserve to be treated with less respect than others. This

is more likely to happen in middle childhood in schools or neighborhoods where there is less diversity and less inclusivity.

Bullying peaks as kids grow older and enter middle school, at about the age of eleven and ending at age fourteen.

According to the National Education Association (NEA), one in three students report being bullied weekly, resulting in serious adverse educational consequences. Students who are targets often experience extreme stress that can lead to symptoms of physical illness and a diminished ability to learn. This translates into increased absenteeism and impaired performance, as indicated by decreased test scores. Educators share that kids report being bullied for reasons based on their weight (23 percent), gender (20 percent), perceived sexual orientation (18 percent), and disability (12 percent). Girls and boys are about equal in being victims of bullying during the school-age years.

It is estimated that over one hundred thousand US children miss school every day due to fear of attack or intimidation by other students. In addition to decreased attendance and poorer academic performance, bullying causes feelings of helplessness, low self-esteem, anger, and fear. In fact, bullying at any age impacts children's mental health and sense of safety, and it's linked to higher rates of social anxiety disorder, depression, and body dysmorphic disorder, and in some extreme cases, trauma.

The consequences aren't limited solely to the person who is bullied. Bullying causes mental harm not only to the victim, but to the bully and the witnesses as well, and research has shown this can persist well into adulthood. A study published in *The Lancet* found that being bullied by peers in childhood had generally worse long-term adverse effects on young adults' mental health than other forms of abuse in childhood. The research team studied the odds of developing mental health problems linked to childhood maltreatment (such as physical, sexual, or emotional abuse) and the odds linked to bullying. They found that bullied children were around five times more likely to experience anxiety and nearly twice as likely to report depression and self-harm at age eighteen than other maltreated children.

These findings have important implications. We need more program development for dealing with peer bullying starting with educating teachers and all school staff on signs of bullying, the law and procedure for reporting, how to talk to children about their experience, and how to support the victim, witnesses, and the bully. Teachers play a critical role in identifying the signs of bullying, protecting children who are victimized, speaking with the families about the incidents, communicating with other school administration, as well as managing the witnesses. However, when studied, nearly half of teachers report they don't know what to do about bullying and lack the adequate knowledge or training in this area.

A key recommendation is that teachers understand how to ask the right questions about events that they suspect may be bullying. There's literature out that says that the way adults ask children questions about bullying can sometimes imply that the child being bullied is somehow to blame or that this child could have done something to cause the bullying. When this occurs, children are much less likely to report bullying and often feel revictimized, confused, and isolated.

How to Help Prevent Your Child from *Being* the Bully

When you think about bullying you probably think of your child in the role of the bullied rather than the bully. You likely don't want to believe that your sweet child is capable of bullying, but I believe it's important for every parent to practice what we know to be effective strategies for bullying *prevention*, including age-appropriate social skills and conflict-resolution techniques, so that *no one's child grows up to be a bully*. These skills not only aim to prevent your child from bullying others, but they will also help you to raise humans who practice empathy and kindness.

In sociology, there's a bias called the "empathy gap," which refers to the block individuals sometimes have in understanding and feeling what someone else is experiencing. Imagine a school playground where a kid is being teased or purposefully excluded by the kids in the class. To those not directly involved, the situation might not seem like too big of a deal, but for the child being bullied, it can be deeply hurtful and isolating. Those witnessing these events might not fully grasp the child's emotional pain, the fear and harassment the bullied child is feeling. Even parents and other adults might underestimate the impact of a bully's words or the lack of action on the part of others to step in. They may not understand the seriousness of the situation or downplay it. This is an empathy gap, and we need to close it.

When I talk about closing the empathy gap, this is a call to action for everyone—students, teachers, and parents alike—to better understand and share in the feelings of those who are being bullied or mistreated in any way. One of the most powerful things you can do as a parent is to check yourself for evidence of an empathy gap. Were you ever bullied or mistreated as a child? Did you ever witness bullying? If so, did you ever do anything about it? Were you ever the bully?

People who have experiences with certain issues, for instance bullying, are more likely to show empathy for others who are going through something similar. On the other hand, if you haven't ever been through bullying, it may be hard for you to appreciate what a child may be experiencing and therefore you may not be responsive or helpful.

Imagine if adults and other children alike could step into the shoes of the child being bullied, even just for that moment. What if everyone could feel the sting of harsh words, the agony of being excluded, and the anxiety of facing another day at school. With this understanding, kids and adults might just be more likely to stand up against bullying, while responding with compassion when they see it, creating a safer environment that would be free of aggression.

The good news is that you can actively teach your kid to be more empathetic. Building empathy is considered one of the more effective tools for instilling a sense of compassion and kindness toward others in kids. This means encouraging your child to listen and learn from others, reflecting on how they would feel in similar situations. It means guiding and modeling for your child what it means to practice acts of kindness. By nurturing empathy, our kids stand a chance to support one another and to help make bullying a thing of the past. Kids and adults of any age can benefit from these conversations.

Here are my tips for bullying prevention:

- Teach your child to use his imagination to think about things from another's perspective. Ask him to imagine how another person might feel about a certain situation. Model empathy by talking about your concern for others, or how you imagine they may be feeling. Read books about characters who go through struggles and challenges and talk about how those situations made the characters feel.
- Teach your children problem-solving skills that are key for their ability to deal with social pressure at this age. This can help prevent them from getting to the point where they feel as if they need to be a bully. When it comes to problem-solving, there's a saying: *you need to name it to tame it*. Teach your child to identify the problem first, then to brainstorm solutions through strategies like a pros and cons lists. You can also encourage your child to first seek guidance from a trusted adult or peer.
- Practice how to resolve disagreements peacefully with your child. Teaching them communication skills such as "I feel ___ when you ___" is a good place to start. They can be reflective listeners; learning how to repeat back what they heard the other person say to be sure they are understanding them correctly can be learned in these middle years. They should also be taught how to give a proper apology and practice forgiving others.
- Give your child plenty of time for unstructured play with peers. This may seem counterintuitive, but if you are worried your child has poor anger-management skills, you can allow her more time to play. When children play, they will learn to recognize and interpret social signals, such as body language and tone of voice, as well as learn to take turns and be more cooperative, all of which are crucial for problem-solving and resolving conflicts with others.

School Anxiety and Avoidance

A few years ago, I treated a fifth-grade boy named Alex with school refusal. His mother reported that the refusal had started as a result of Alex going to overnight camp in the summer and becoming extremely homesick. Alex would call almost nightly crying and saying that he wanted to come home. But as his parents felt it would be best for him to stick it out, he had spent fourteen days waking up anxious and tired from not sleeping well, having a fairly fun time throughout the day, and then suffering from stomachaches, not eating well, and crying himself to sleep at night. When August rolled around and it was time to start his new middle school, Alex started reporting very bad stomachaches, dizzy spells, or headaches. His first day of school his mom had to pick him up around lunchtime. Then the following days Alex would either get on the bus crying or had to be driven in late or picked up early, and by October he was missing school two to three days a week. That's when the parents called me.

Alex's parents shared with me that they had no idea what to do with their son, who was only managing a few days a week at school—the other days, the panic was too severe for him to move. "He has a stomachache or headaches every day," the parents explained. "The night before school he wants us to lie with him in bed until he falls asleep, and usually, he wakes up in the middle of the night with a nightmare. We talk about ideas of what can help him, but they don't seem to work, and we don't know what else to do." A few weeks before we met, Child Protective Services (CPS) was called on this family due to the number of missed school days. When the social worker asked the child why he wasn't going to school, Alex said that his brain was telling him that he should go but his body felt it was too much, his legs began to shake, his heart started to pound, and the sensations of wanting to vomit took over.

It's notable that this started happening during the transition from fifth-grade elementary school to sixth-grade middle school. School refusal is often seen during times of transition, either from elementary to middle, or middle to high school. In this respect, it's actually quite similar to preschool separation anxiety, when kids don't want to leave their parent to go to nursery school or daycare. School avoidance also tends to be a gradual process; it doesn't happen overnight. Kids start with missing a day here and there, then missing a week, which leads to another week, until the student becomes school avoidant altogether. The more time a student is away from school, the harder it is to get him back into school, and if a parent works from home, it's easier to justify that the kid can just stay home. Since the pandemic, this is a cycle that many parents have found themselves trapped in.

School refusal typically has a root cause of anxiety. Children with school refusal may experience severe emotional distress at the thought of going to school, like Alex, which can lead to panic attacks. This distress can have physical symptoms (like nausea or headaches) or behavioral symptoms (such as tantrums or defiance). Some kids who struggle with school refusal will miss school several days a week or may call home to leave early on a frequent basis or find places to escape—namely the nurse's office or a school counselor's office. A child's intense worry related to school can include fear of failure, social anxiety with peers, or general anxiety about attending school. I see this starting as young as kindergarten and it can span through elementary school.

The effects of school refusal run deep. The child is stressed, grades suffer, and there's a greater risk they won't graduate. The whole family is stressed, with parents describing it as a never-ending sense of dread and worry. Socially, these kids struggle because they aren't in school, they aren't maintaining friendships, and typically they don't do many, if any, activities outside of their home. All these combined compromises their overall well-being.

Since spring 2020, schools have closed, then reopened, then partially opened, then quarantined, then opened again, but still today too many students don't regularly attend school. To be considered high in absenteeism a child would have to miss 10 percent or more of the school year, equivalent to about eighteen days of school. The latest numbers estimate that chronic absenteeism is still *double the rate* of pre-pandemic figures. In 2023, one in four students were chronically absent. According to the US Department of Education, prior to the pandemic, it used to be one in five. Of course, not all absences from school are due to school refusal. A child may be physically unwell or have family caretaking obligations. They may simply skip school or sleep in too late. Not all absences are necessarily linked to anxiety or fear, but school refusal cases may have also grown as students report experiencing anxiety at record levels. A Kaiser Family Foundation analysis found adolescents experiencing anxiety or depression increased by one-third from 2016 to 2020. The same report also found access to mental health services worsened during the pandemic. As school refusal is considered a symptom of anxiety, treatment for the child is important as well as support for parents who often feel shamed and blamed.

What to Do If Your Child Is Struggling with School Anxiety

If your child is experiencing anxiety around school, this can affect the whole family. Mornings can be a minefield, with your anxious child struggling even to walk to the school bus stop or get in the car with a parent. Tears may start, protest begins, or panic sets in. As a parent you may also break out in tears, argue with your child, and negotiate with him, even offering bribes. But after a while, you realize that this isn't going anywhere.

I often get calls from parents when they are in the thick of it. The first thing I advise is that they calm themselves first and then approach their child with an openness to hearing anything that child has to share.

Here are some dos and don'ts if your child is struggling with school anxiety:

- Do talk to your child as calmly as you can. Don't counterargue or disagree with something your child tells you, just listen and take it in. Find moments to talk to your child about the avoidance that aren't in the morning or at bedtime, when everyone is either rushing or tired.
- Do acknowledge how hard it is for him to go to school. Don't dismiss him or tell him that he "just needs to go to school. Period."
- Do send your child the message that you are in it together by getting to his level, with a supportive stance and reassurance that this won't last forever. This may not help your child reduce anxiety that very day, but it will help him to feel like his parent is no longer angry at him and instead that you are aligning with him to come up with a solution.
- Do try to help your child to figure out his triggers, the people, places, or aspects of school that may be causing his distress. It could be a teacher, a certain classmate, a particular time of the day (like lunch), or even a subject like PE. If he says he doesn't know, be patient, ask him to pretend to know—to guess. This tends to calm the situation.
- Don't try to come up with solutions until you have an understanding of the underlying causes of the worry or avoidance. Anxiety is typically the main underlying cause, but there are also situations that can involve bullying or learning challenges at school that a child is actively trying to

avoid. Your child may have sensory challenges around classroom noise or an uncomfortable uniform that's causing him distress. You won't know what's really bothering your child until you ask the questions and listen for the answers.

- Do create a plan. Once you have a better idea of underlying causes, you need to come up with a plan that entails setting clear expectations for your child. You can tell your child that you are going to work with him and with his school to address the things that are worrying him. You can explain that going to school is very important and that the goal is for him to attend without feeling so much stress and worry anymore.
- Do establish calming routines at night and in the morning. Even though your child is older now, he will still benefit from the kinds of simple routines that helped him to settle down and get out of the door when he was a preschooler. You can even have a chart that shows the sequence for bedtime and mornings pinned to the wall.
- Do stay in close communication with your child's school. One thing that can be helpful is to track your child's anxiety to see if there are patterns. Be clear and upfront with the school about what he's experiencing and what you are doing to help him. If absenteeism is becoming an issue, reach out to your child's pediatrician or psychologist for help and documentation. This can help avoid the school administration becoming reactive and calling in outside agencies if your child misses an excessive amount of school.
- Do understand that helping your child move beyond school anxiety can take time. When I'm working with families dealing with school avoidance, I typically start with what we call gradual exposure, which means systematically reintroducing the child to the school environment. This may include starting with shorter days or specific classes and increasing the amount of time until the child can tolerate a full school day. This is made possible by creating a supportive environment in collaboration with administration and teachers at school.
- Do find a trusted adult or friend at school who can help your child in the school setting. Is there a favorite teacher who can be at the school door to greet your child and help him with the transition to the classroom? Or a buddy who will walk with him to the bus in the mornings? These relationships can help lower your child's cortisol levels and can be key to helping him regulate again at school.

Active Shooter Drills in School

I started my doctoral program the year after the Columbine shooting and currently live just two miles away from the school. Every single day I am reminded of the countless ways that schools have changed since that tragic day in 1999. One of the many changes that affects children in middle childhood is their awareness of school shootings as well as their experiences with active shooter drills. Remember when you used to have fire drills in grade school? I am guessing that this isn't a scary memory for you because you had likely never seen or experienced a fire in a school. But today, active shooter drills, designed to prepare students and staff for potential school shootings, have become a common practice in many schools across the US. While the purpose behind these drills is to improve safety, they can have significant psychological and emotional impacts on school-age children.

Active shooter drills can induce significant anxiety and fear among kids. The experience of these drills, and lockdowns, which can include simulating the sounds of gunfire and having students practice hiding or barricading doors, can be highly distressing. Young children and teens alike may have difficulty distinguishing between a drill and a real threat, leading to what some kids have described as "traumatic" experiences.

The psychological effects of these drills can be profound and long-lasting. Repeated exposure to simulated threats, especially without warning or clarity that they are only drills, can contribute to a sense of vulnerability and helplessness. The constant reminder of the potential for a school shooting can also wear away at their sense of safety.

The impact of active shooter drills and lockdowns extends beyond immediate anxiety and fear. These drills can affect students' overall well-being. The stress associated with these drills can exacerbate existing mental health issues, such as trauma, anxiety, and depression.

Drills and lockdowns impact the whole school environment. Kids look at other kids' backpacks and wonder what's in them. Teachers and staff, too, are impacted by the toll of practicing these drills and managing their own fears of what-ifs. Teachers have shared that they think about their own death, and they question their ability to keep a whole classroom safe and alive.

In order to mitigate this stress, schools should provide assurance to their community that by practicing these drills it helps to prevent a tragedy from happening and offer support for students who find them distressing. Schools should also always inform parents when they happen so parents can discuss it with their kids. Involving mental health professionals in the planning and execution of these drills can help ensure that they are done in a way that minimizes harmful impacts.

Pressure and Sports

I first started seeing Jay when he was eleven years old for a referral of sports-related anxiety. When I met with the family Jay was just starting middle school and was at the highest level in travel club baseball for his age. He was already known locally throughout the state, as was his father, who was a former professional athlete. The increased attention Jay was getting for his pitching was starting to get distracting, and his parents thought I could help with Jay's focus and regulation. Since my expertise is in anxiety disorders, I will see athletes who are wanting to work on adrenaline management, anxiety control, and mental strength.

Jay and I worked together right up until high school started. Over the course of two years, we addressed issues around focus, visualization, breathing, rest, and managing the pressure he felt from his father. Our work included family sessions with Jay's dad, who was fairly receptive to feedback. Over time, his father learned that coaching from the stands wasn't helping Jay, neither was dissecting each game on the car ride home. Instead, he needed to be present and supportive of his son. Jay's siblings talked about how they were tired of always being at baseball games and how they wished they traveled less and did more as a family. The parents did their best to empathize with the younger siblings and started splitting travel time instead of all always going to Jay's games.

We wrapped up our work as Jay was starting at a high school where he liked the coach and where they thought he had the best chance of success. I wished him the best as we said goodbye and told him I would be here for him should he need a little "tune-up" along the way. I knew he had made lots of strides and that I might see him again, maybe as he got more playing time in high school or during the travel season for his club team where the pressure was sure to increase. In the spring of sophomore year, I got a call from Jay's dad saying that he wanted me to work with Jay again. Apparently, the night before, Jay had told his parents he was "burned out" and wanted to quit playing. While this came as a surprise for Jay's parents, sadly, it didn't for me.

According to a 2024 report from the AAP, 70 percent of children drop out of sports by the age of thirteen. Kids report that it is around this age that sports become less fun and less social. It goes from *playing* a game to *competing* in a sport. The age of thirteen or right before is the time when kids typically get split into different teams by ability; sometimes they are traveling and sometimes they simply don't make the cut. For a majority of athletes, the numbers speak for themselves: they simply quit. Between multiple days a week of training, pressure to choose a single sport to focus on, and overuse injuries, kids burn out right at about thirteen which means they are only in seventh or eighth grade. They aren't even out of middle school yet.

And if they do make it out of middle school still involved in a sport, the pressure really increases as talk of playing at a collegiate level starts to mount. I remember Kiki, one girl I worked with, who had picked up volleyball in middle school. It started off as fun and social for playing on her school team with friends, and then in eighth grade she decided to start playing for a club to get better. The summer before her freshman year in high school, Kiki showed up for summer practices, attended clinics, and endured a two-day tryout only to not even make the team. The school she had chosen to attend was filled with girls aspiring to play volleyball in college, and they all had much more experience and club play than she had. At the age of fourteen, Kiki was done with sports.

Stories like these happen all across America each year. Kids don't make teams, or they don't play or get cut as new and better athletes crowd the roster. Kids who want to play are either left with no options or they feel downgraded to recreational (rec) teams, which can carry stigma for kids who want to identify as a stronger athlete. There is a divide between competitive and rec teams starting as young as ten years old. According to the AAP, discontinuation of sports during childhood plays a role in the more than 75 percent of US adolescents failing to meet physical activity recommendations.

And what about those kids who do get picked for the competitive teams? A 2024 AAP report made updates to their prior report, adding "considerable evidence to better define how excessive training volumes can lead to overuse injury, overtraining, impaired well-being, and decreased quality of life." So, on the one hand the kids who stick with sports might be overtraining and getting injured, while the other kids are shut out and not physically active. None of these eventualities are good for developing children. And unfortunately, neighborhood pickup games seem to be a thing of the past—even though that's exactly what many of today's youth need—a variety of sports that they can play with friends and other kids for fun after school and on weekends just for bragging rights.

The physical and psychological benefits for kids who play team sports seem to last through to adulthood. A study published in the *Journal of Adolescent Health* found that students who play team sports in grades eight through twelve have less stress and better mental health as young adults. Specifically, physical activity reduces the levels of the stress hormone cortisol. It also releases endorphins, the "feel good" hormones. It also increases serotonin, a chemical that plays an important role in mood. Socially, being on a team creates a sense of belonging, which can result in positive self-esteem, connection with peers, and confidence. Many of us have experienced that even one hour of physical activity helps reduce stress and anxiety, as well as create feelings of well-being for several hours after exercising. In other words, regularly playing a variety of organized team sports may be an overlooked protective factor in the youth mental health crisis.

Team sport participation is thought to be particularly effective in protecting against the development of mental health problems among children and adolescents because of the many opportunities for connection through team belonging. Human beings are wired for connection: we need it, or we die. This is a way to get that for your child while also reaping the physical health benefits and all that comes along with it. "Participation in youth team sports has been linked with lower rates of depression and anxiety, along with a reduced risk of suicide and substance abuse," says Soroosh Amanat, MD, a family medicine physician in sports medicine. One study of teens with depression found that the effects of exercise actually lasted longer than those of antidepressants and therapy.

According to a 2022 study, children who are involved in sports between the ages of eight and ten years old had more positive health-related quality of life scores and lower rates of psychological challenges at age ten as compared with children who stopped playing sports by age ten. Kids who participated in team sports compared to kids who did not participate were associated with 10 percent lower anxious/depressed scores, 19 percent lower withdrawn/depressed scores, 17 percent lower social problems scores, 17 percent lower thought problems scores, and 12 percent lower attention problems scores. Results indicate that *team* sport participation was associated with fewer mental health difficulties, whereas *individual* sport participation was associated with greater mental health difficulties. The findings are consistent with previous research suggesting that team sport participation may be a tool to support child and adolescent mental health under two unique conditions: when participation is established between the ages of eight to ten and when it's participation in team sport versus an individual sport. This doesn't mean your child can't do an individual sport (my own kids play tennis, rock climb, and run) but having at least one team sport for part of the year has been shown to have significant benefits.

Being involved in team sports is also associated with higher academic achievement in high school students. Possible explanations for this relationship between participation in team sports and better academic performance include a student's sense of identity with school sports and the associated school culture and values, which could, in turn, improve the students' academic performance. Further, team sports participation can strengthen the athlete's psychological resilience, self-esteem, self-discipline, and overall life skills. These skills have been recognized as incentives to better academic performance.

Dr. Amanat also points out that more time spent playing sports means less time on social media. And as kids get older, many coaches are monitoring and advising around social media posts, warning athletes that some posts could cost them interest or even offers from schools if it isn't in line with their values. Looking ahead, if you have an athlete, sharing this with them, as well as pointing to high-profile stories in which it actually happened, will be an important lesson. Being involved in team sports represents an important avenue for lifelong physical activity that is key to physical and mental health.

One promising trend in youth sports is a new push for mental health literacy to be a part of organized sports. One study of a sports-based mental health intervention for boys aged twelve to eighteen showed that the group who was offered the intervention showed improvements in signs and symptoms of depression and anxiety, and also gave them a greater desire to help those struggling with mental health issues. This is proving to be particularly helpful for boys who may be socialized to think they can't talk about feelings or seek help if they're struggling emotionally.

But while we wait for more of these programs to be included in schools and sports leagues, you will want to find ways of including sports as a part of your child's life without falling prey to the pressure. My message to parents is: don't be surprised if your child is struggling with a high-pressure sports environment or talking about dropping out. Instead, work with your child to find ways for him to participate in team sports without the pressure—whether that means playing pickup games at the park, finding a rec league, or even organizing a local team of your own with friends and where the focus is on team building and fun.

Looking Ahead

At some point in the next couple of years, your child is going to want to try all kinds of different activities, sports-related or otherwise. Keep options open instead of being rigid about what you think your child should or shouldn't do. When children are constantly pushed to meet high expectations, they may develop a fear of failure, leading to avoidance, reducing their intrinsic motivation, and halting their potential. This pressure can also damage their self-esteem and strain parent-child relationships. Get ready to go from the director of your child's sports choices, activities, or relationships to supportive guide.

In a Nutshell

Before you know it, your child is going to be preparing for entry to high school, and then for college. If you exert too much pressure on your child to succeed now—whether academically or athletically—you run the risk of burnout before he even makes it to college. Instead, you need to balance your expectations of your child with plenty of time for free play, socializing, creative pursuits, and time with you. Here's a summary of the many ways to help your child succeed in life without undue pressure.

- Prioritize your child's mental health over his academic/sports success.
- Give your child more autonomy, allowing him to develop a sense of mastery.
- Praise your child sparingly and specifically.
- Give your child chores and opportunities to make money.
- Value kindness in your child.
- Help your child develop organizational skills to deal with his school load.
- Stay alert for bullying and take action whether your child is being bullied or bullying.
- Teach your child empathy, social skills, and communication.
- Help your child to identify and talk about emotions.
- If your child is struggling with school avoidance, collaborate with your child and his school to identify triggers and to mitigate them.
- Serve as your child's guide and support system, not his drillmaster.
- Find ways for your child to participate in and enjoy team sports without a high degree of pressure.

CHAPTER 6

Understanding Sexual and Gender Identity Development

Maybe... I am learning from my brave son.

—Mr. Effiong from the show *Sex Education* on Netflix

When I was approaching puberty back in the late 1980s, I never would have *dreamed* of going to my mom to talk about sex, sexuality, or anything to do with my developing sense of myself as a young woman. I didn't speak to her about these touchy subjects, and she didn't speak about them either. Instead, I put together bits and pieces of information from different sources: from my friends and their older sisters, from Judy Blume books, and from whispers under the covers at sleepover parties. I was definitely the girl in my bedroom chanting "I must, I must, I must increase my bust," who stuffed her bra, and sometimes even slept in it because I thought it would keep my breasts firm. It was a given that I was heterosexual, that my identity was female, and there were zero messages around any other way to be. As a kid, it felt like I was on a mystery journey of my own to figure how I felt about being a young woman and my sexuality. Like a *Scooby-Doo* episode, the journey was a little scary, but in the end, I figured it would all work out. I don't remember if I wished someone would talk about these things with me: I didn't know any different, and my friends were in the same boat. I just remember I had a lot of questions and a sense of being on a solo mission to figure things out.

Times, as they say, have definitely changed. Since I began teaching my Start with the Talk classes in 2013, I have met with hundreds of young girls and their parents to talk about all things puberty. But of all the topics we tackle in this class, it's gender and sexual development that generate the most questions, the majority of them coming, not from the kids, but from the adults. This is a subject that confuses many parents of Generation Alpha kids (born 2010 to the present). These parents are mostly Millennials (born between 1981 and 1996) of whom around 10 percent identify as LGBTQ+.[1]

Children today are growing up in a world where the language around sexual identity has widened far beyond heterosexual, gay, lesbian, and bisexual to include asexual (not interested in sex or romance), demisexual (feels sexual attraction only when they've established an emotional bond with someone), and pansexual (can feel sexual attraction to anyone regardless of their gender or sexuality), and more.[2] Meanwhile, increasing numbers of young people are identifying outside of the gender binary of male and female, across a spectrum of fluidity that's confusing to many cisgender parents ("cis" means your internal sense of gender matches the gender you were assigned at birth).

What I've learned from spending time with families in my practice is that the *kids* are already quite well-informed on issues to do with sexuality and gender.[3] Despite the fact that many states don't mandate sex education at any age, with only a small number of states requiring medically accurate information if sex ed is on the curriculum, many kids at this age are actually fairly comfortable talking about these issues. Thanks to a surge in awareness and access to information online, they've grown up understanding terms that weren't even on their parents' radar at the same age. Instead, it tends to be the parents who feel lost and unable to navigate this landscape. This, for me, is the biggest change from when I was growing up. Back then, kids were the ones who were confused. Now, it's the parents who are more confused!

In my course, the kids' questions on gender and sexuality usually take the form of "How do you know if you like your friend as a friend, or if it's a crush?" or "What if I don't know yet if I like boys or girls?" The parents' questions are about how to understand their children as their kids figure out who they like, how they identify, and how they want to dress to reflect that. Here's a sampling:

- Since when did ten-year-olds start wearing crop tops? Is this okay?
- What age is it okay to let my daughter have a boyfriend? And if they don't really do anything, does it really count?
- My son rates girls' looks and talks to his friends about their hotness scores. He is a seventh-grade boy, but this all feels too fast to me. What should I say to him?
- My son has become a lot more private lately in his room and his bathroom, but his younger sisters still go into his room without knocking. How do I explain to them why their brother needs so much privacy all of a sudden?
- My son told me he's gay. I know his life is going to be so much harder now. Is this something I should really support when I know he is more likely to be bullied or suffer from depression?
- How do I know if my kid is really gay/trans/nonbinary or if it's just a phase? He's still so young. How can he really know? Can he grow out of it?

The reality is that Gen Alpha kids are going to be exposed to a much wider range of ways to identify and present themselves than you were, which can leave you without much personal experience to fall back on at this stage of their lives. In my sessions, many parents have no idea how to talk to their child who may be using terms they don't understand like "cisgender." When I ask their child to explain, parents sometimes ask me if these words have been made up.

Reading this, you may question whether your elementary or middle school child is old enough to have any understanding of these issues yet. You may worry about whether or not you may "influence" your child in some way by engaging with them about these topics. You may be concerned that you're going to create confusion in your child by introducing them to "adult" information. In fact, this is a crucial developmental period in children's lives when their sexual and gender identities may be in flux. If there's one thing I want you to take away from this chapter, it's that this kind of development is *absolutely normal* and natural at this age. The way you have these conversations with your child today can have a significant impact on the conversations you're able to have later, and on them developing a strong sense of self as they grow.

Sound Familiar?

- Your six-year-old boy sometimes wants to play with his sister's dolls, and you feel a ping of anxiety inside.
- You keep telling yourself you will get around to talking to your kid about crushes and relationships, but you never seem to find the right time.
- You looked through your kid's phone or tablet and saw that they have been searching up sexual terms, but you don't know how to talk to them about it.
- Your kid has been through some sex education at school, you asked them about it, and they said it was "fine" or "boring." You're not sure if you should ask them again about it or just move on—if they have questions they can ask you.
- Your child hasn't had any sex education at school yet, and so you don't want to broach this topic with them before his teachers do.
- Messages like "boys can wear pink and cry" and "girls can do and be anything" have you questioning how you would even know if your child had issues; it seems like anything goes these days.

PARADIGM SHIFT

Paradigm: My kid is too young to think about or talk about sexuality and gender. I don't want to upset them or give them ideas by talking to them about these issues. We can have these discussions *if* they come up when they're older.

Shift: Your child is already thinking about and talking about sexuality and gender with their peers, and you definitely want to get involved in these conversations, which will likely be much more complex than the ones you had when you were their age.

Sexual Identity

UNDERSTANDING SEXUAL DEVELOPMENT IN CHILDREN

Sexual development is the process through which kids experience physical, emotional, and psychological changes related to their sexuality. This phase of development encompasses various aspects, including biological changes, sexual orientation, gender identity, and the development of healthy relationships. During middle childhood, children are going through hormonal changes that are, essentially, preparing the body for potential reproduction, including breast development and menstruation in girls and the enlarging of the penis and testes in boys. But children are also going through major shifts in their awareness of sexuality in general. Your child may begin to experience attraction and they may start to have crushes. All of a sudden, they may become uncomfortable around a friend they've known for years, without understanding why. They may find that their crushes are directed toward people of the opposite gender (heterosexuality) or the same gender (homosexuality).

You may think back fondly to the times when your son played house with a little girl in his preschool class, pretending to be the dad while she pretended to be the mom. Back then, they were engaging in socialized play—which is play that mimics the roles children see around them. Now that they're approaching the pubertal phase, it's typical for children to begin to figure out who they might be attracted to in terms of romantic relationships. They may have known when they were younger, but in puberty, this feeling tends to become more definitive.[4]

One of the things that happens at this crucial age is that parents clam up and fail to have conversations around sexuality in any shape or form. On the one hand, children start to become aware of attraction and sexual orientation—and they certainly begin to talk about it with peers. And on the other hand, parents feel uncomfortable, so they wind up not saying anything! This leads children to believe that these topics are off-limits. If your child isn't talking to you about this, it may mean that they aren't thinking about this yet, or it may mean they've taken your silence to mean they *can't* talk about this with you.

At this age, the main way kids will think about sexuality is through the frame of "crushes." Some kids are very open about talking to their parents about their crushes. Others aren't inclined to talk at all. If your child does come to you to tell you they have a crush or to ask about feelings of attraction they might have to another child, whatever you do, don't dismiss them. Don't say, "You're too young to think about that!" Kids can have crushes as early as preschool; it's part of their development. Instead, you can say, "Oh, tell me about that. What makes you feel that way?"

Sometimes children will ask, "How do I know it's a crush and I don't want just to be friends with that person?" When a child in my practice asks me this question I say, "When it's a crush you might get butterflies in your stomach when you see them, you might think about them a lot, you might doodle their name in your notebook." When talking to children about crushes, I always reinforce that it's important to feel *good* around somebody you like, to feel you're yourself around that person. "You should spend time with people who make you feel good about yourself" is a really helpful message to send to your child at this age.

Other times, your child may be unsure about whether they have feelings for a friend who is the same sex and what that means. If your child comes to you because they're feeling confused, you can say, "So right now you're really questioning how you feel about different people. We don't have to define anything yet if you don't want to. This is what you're supposed to be doing at this age—your brain is asking so many questions. Feelings can come and go and sometimes you don't know why, and that's okay too."

If your child doesn't bring up the subject with you directly, there are ways to open up the conversation:

- Start with your observations. "I noticed that you're trying on a new look . . ." "I noticed you don't see so much of your oldest friend anymore . . ." "I noticed you have some new friends . . ."
- Answer your child's questions truthfully (within reason). They may ask about your first crush or your how old you were when you first dated.
- Watch the shows and videos that they're watching and talk about them with them. That's how you can stay connected and tap into where they are with their interests and identity.

- Talk openly about the three basic sexual orientations with your child: same sex (gay and lesbian), opposite sex (heterosexual), and both sexes (bisexual). As we've observed, there are many more labels, but for ages six to twelve it may be enough to start with these three.

Sexual Orientation in Children

- For a long time, social scientists believed that very young kids didn't have the cognitive ability to understand sexual orientation. But that attitude is changing. Kids are potentially considering their sexuality and learning about themselves at a younger age than previously thought. The reality is that many kids know they are gay (or not) younger than you might expect—even in elementary school. One study by San Diego State University surveyed thousands of youth across the nation. They found that 1 percent of kids ages nine to ten identify as gay, bisexual, or transgender.
- Many children and adults in my class ask me the same question: "Are kids 'born this way' like Lady Gaga sings about?" If your child asks you this question, you can answer simply: yes. Being straight, gay, or bisexual is not something that a child chooses. In fact, kids don't choose their sexual orientation any more than they choose their height or eye color. You can also explain to your child that people who identify as LGBTQ+ come from all ethnicities, religions, and socioeconomic groups.
- No one fully understands exactly what determines a person's sexual orientation, but it is likely explained by a mix of biological and genetic factors. Organizations such as the American Academy of Pediatrics (AAP) and the American Psychological Association (APA) view sexual orientation as part of someone's nature. Being gay is also not considered a mental disorder or abnormality (although it used to be until 1973).
- Despite decades of theories, there is no evidence that being gay is caused by early childhood experiences, parenting styles, or the way someone was raised. And there appears to be no such thing as a single gay gene either. The authors of a 2019 study[5] analyzed half a million people and concluded that genetics has a limited contribution to sexual orientation. They could

not find a gene that says, "Yes, you're gay." And so, we still don't have a clear picture of the biological causes involved. What we do know is that efforts to "change" gay people from homosexual to heterosexual (historically called "conversion therapy") have been proven to be ineffective and can be extremely harmful. The majority of reputable mental health professionals caution against any efforts to change a person's sexual orientation.

- While most social scientists agree that children are born with a certain sexual orientation, this doesn't mean this orientation is always set in stone. Middle childhood marks the beginning of a child's understanding of his sexuality, and this may necessarily be a time of flux for them—and that's normal. This truth about a child's development can be extremely confusing and upsetting for some parents. I remember one parent coming to me because her eight-year-old son Jason had told her that he wanted to marry a boy. Her reaction was, "You're eight years old! You don't know what you want yet! Why are you even saying that?" In our parent session that same week, she wanted to know if it was possible her son really *was* gay. "Could he really know at this age?" I said, "I don't know. He's at an age where this kind of exploration is normal. What *I* know for certain is that when he came to you, he wanted to know what *your* reaction would be. The most important thing you can do right now is to tell him that it's okay, that he's at an age where he's figuring out a lot of stuff, including who he might have feelings toward, and that's normal."
- My message for parents with children this age who seem to be exploring who they're attracted to is meet your child where they are. Don't impose your own fears or expectations on your child. Allow your child the space to ask questions, explore, and grow. This is what children are supposed to be doing at this age.
- Many parents are concerned that if they talk about different sexual orientations, they will influence their children to "become gay." They point to the increasing numbers of children who are identifying as LGBTQ+ and they say this is because we're allowing and encouraging this "lifestyle choice." Many parents ask me, "When do we step in as adults and say this is too much?" I do not have one blanket answer for these parents, and I can't dictate to them whether or not their child's orientation aligns with their values or not. What I can do is to give parents' permission to be open and say, "Let's talk about this," rather than shutting down the

conversation. Maybe your child is going through a phase, and they will "grow into a new one," or maybe they aren't. School-age children are old enough to know if they're gay or not. In fact, a 2013 Pew Research Center study shows that 59 percent of gay kids say they knew between the ages of ten and nineteen that they were gay, and 24 percent said they knew before the age of ten.[6] We may not know if your child's crush is a passing stage or an indication of future sexual orientation, but it's important to recognize that both scenarios are normal and not to discount your child's feelings.

- If your kid tells you they are gay, you *can say*, "You're figuring out who you are and that's normal for your age. I am glad you are comfortable telling me, I love you no matter who you love!" Remember, if your child shares something like this with you and you don't know what to say; you can always tell him "Thank you for trusting me enough to share this with me. I don't know exactly what to say right now except that I love you and nothing can ever change that." When you show sensitivity and acceptance, your child will trust you, and this means they will come to you for support in the future—how you respond can also make a crucial difference in your child's future mental health and self-esteem. More on this below.

Teaching Your Child to be an Ally

The middle childhood years are a good time to talk to your child about being an ally or upstander to their LGBTQ+ peers. You can explain to them that being an ally means "helping or supporting other people who are part of a group that is treated badly or unfairly, although you are not yourself a member of this group."[7] The reality is you're much more likely to influence an eight-year-old than you are a fourteen- or fifteen-year-old boy who has grown accustomed to using "gay" as a slur or who ribs others in his peer group for being too effeminate. When you tell an eight-year-old "that's not the way we talk in this family or how we treat people," your child is more likely to internalize that message.

Here are some tips for how to talk about this issue:

- Caution your child against using "gay" as an insult. Explain to him that when he says this, it makes being gay something to be ashamed of, and it shouldn't be. Tell your child "We don't do that" and "Your words matter."
- Explain to your child that one of the most important ways to practice allyship is just to listen with curiosity and without judgment. When you listen, learn, support, and offer acceptance, you're practicing true allyship.
- Explain to your child that if they hear another child bullying or saying things that are derogatory toward others, they should feel empowered to stand up to that bully, or to tell you or another adult.

Mental Health of LGBTQ+ Children

Today, the thinking is that youth who identify as LGBTQ+ are not inherently prone to mental health problems because of their sexual orientation or gender identity. Rather, they often face issues like rejection, bullying, stigmatization, discrimination, and violence that put them at a higher risk of mental health challenges including depression, anxiety, and suicidal feelings. The numbers are a real cause for concern: lesbian, gay, and bisexual youth are more than twice as likely as their heterosexual peers to struggle with feelings of sadness and hopelessness, while trans and gender-diverse youth are more than twice as likely as their peers to experience depression and suicidal feelings.[8] The Trevor Project, a nonprofit that concentrates on suicide prevention efforts among youth who are LGBTQ+, estimates that 1.8 million LGBTQ+ young people seriously consider suicide every year in the US,[9] with at least one attempt every forty-five seconds. Nearly one in five transgender and nonbinary youth has attempted suicide. LGBTQ+ youth of color reported higher rates of suicide attempts than their White peers, and 45 percent of LGBTQ+ youth seriously considered attempting suicide in the past year. And 60 percent of LGBTQ+ youth who wanted mental health care in the past year were unable to get it.

As a parent, your number one concern will always be your child's happiness and safety, but the reality is, you can't always change how others will respond to your child. You *can*, however, reduce the impact of risk factors like bullying, discrimination, and rejection on your child. We call these "protective factors," and they make it less likely that kids will develop mental health challenges.

Here's the number one thing you need to know: the most important protective factor for LGBTQ+ kids is *having unconditional love and support at home*. Other factors include:

- validation, which means that you say, "I see you, I want to support you as you are, I don't want to change you"
- involvement in some sort of group or having friendships with other LGBTQ+ kids or seeking out a mentor
- therapy with an LGBTQ+ affirming therapist can help with processing emotions, coming up with coping skills, and understanding identity. Support groups for kids and parents can offer another protective factor

You may want to believe by ignoring or dismissing your child's sexual or gender identity you can make it "go away." You may hope that your child will grow out of whatever they're feeling now so they won't have to deal with the challenges of growing up in a world that isn't always welcoming or kind to LGBTQ+ people. But in fact, when you embrace your child—meeting them where they're at right now instead of dismissing them—you are actually *protecting them from the harm that can come their way in the future*. Study after study has found that parents who support their LGBTQ+ children can make a real difference in their kid's mental health outcomes. LGBTQ+ youth who felt high social support from their family reported attempting suicide at less than half the rate of those who felt low or moderate social support.[10]

Understanding Relationships and Consent at This Age

During this period in a child's life, they will begin to learn about healthy and sometimes unhealthy relationships. When a child is at the start of puberty, they will begin to explore new friendships, push boundaries at home, and if there are siblings involved, those dynamics may start to shift too. It's important to understand that this is all healthy, normal, and part of child development. Kids will test out relationships at this age, usually with the ones they love and trust the most—parents and siblings—so they can go out and explore these dynamics outside the home with others. They may practice this for years with family and friends before they are ever in a romantic relationship.

When it comes to romantic relationships, kids typically don't start puberty and then immediately start to feel attraction toward others. It can take a while to understand their newfound feelings and then to express them. Once puberty has begun, relationship desires are a normal part of the process.

Around this age, a child begins to learn about the concept of consent. Simply put: consent means when you agree or give permission to another person to do something to you, and it's often used in a sexual context. Your goal is for your child to understand consent *in general* so that when they start to have romantic relationships, they can respect another person's boundaries and make sure that their own boundaries are respected. Although it's a good idea to talk to your child about sexual consent and what that means, you can actually foster this sense of understanding in your daily life through your actions. When you are clear about setting and maintaining boundaries (not using foul language, not taking the phone out at dinner) you are actually showing your child how much they can push the limits in relationships: your child will take their cues from the way parents and other adults respond to them. This is why it's really important to allow your child to give *their* consent on some issues, such as having their picture taken and shared on social media, not having to hug someone if they don't feel comfortable, or respecting their privacy in the bathroom (knock before going in). By giving your child this autonomy, you're actually teaching them about consent.

How to Talk About Sex with Your Child in a Way That's Age Appropriate

As part of sexual development, children seek to understand their own sexuality and that of others. This includes learning about naked bodies and sex. They may even want to know about sexually transmitted diseases and contraception.

I know for many parents this is overwhelming to think about. If you are picturing your sweet nine-year-old daughter or eleven-year-old son searching online for videos to see what sex looks like or googling "What's a good penis size?" you likely want to skip right over this chapter. I get it. But these are not made-up hypothetical situations; both of those examples come from kids I have treated.

Parents often ask me when to have these conversations with children, as most parents are uncomfortable bringing up this topic. Over 20 percent of parents don't plan to bring up sex with their kids at all, and one in four admit they would "feel awkward" talking about sex with their children. Perhaps this isn't surprising. Stop and think right now—did anyone talk to you about sexual identity? How did you find out about sex? Contraception? Abortion? In fact, six out of ten parents in America say they were raised to think sex was a "taboo" subject.[11] I'm pretty sure most of my knowledge came from watching teen movies. No adult ever taught me about these things. It was all social learning from friends, siblings, and shows like *The Facts of Life*. Today, if you don't teach your kids, you risk having your kids research this on their own online or on social media.

While it's important to take the lead on the sex talk, I don't usually advocate for parents to talk about what I consider "older" topics, such as sexually transmitted infections, for example, until children are in their early teens and it's more relevant to them. In my puberty class, which is for girls twelve and under, I focus on teaching children about their growing and changing body, and then at the end of the class I hand each parent a sheet that covers major topics that are necessary to talk about between the ages of twelve and fourteen. This is an ongoing conversation.

Here's my general advice about what to cover and when:

- **From ages four to seven:** Cover the basics of "where babies come from" with your child. You should also talk about boundaries and private parts, that no one is allowed to look at their private parts or to touch them—and if this happens that they must tell a parent or another adult right away.
- **From ages seven to twelve:** My advice is to focus mainly on building on what you have already covered and then addressing identity development, identity expression, and puberty.

- **Ages twelve and up:** You should plan to have conversations around issues such as sexual consent, sexually transmitted infections, sexual assault, contraception, abortion, and pregnancy. You may decide to introduce these topics earlier or later depending on how quickly your child seems to be progressing toward having romantic relationships and generally what they have been exposed to.

Some families are very open about having these conversations at younger ages, and others never have the talk at all. No matter where you fall on that spectrum, I want parents to think of this as *a trajectory*. Even if you start with the stork, you need to progress and step up the information you're giving your child as they grow and mature.

The Importance of Talking to Your Child About Pornography

In today's world, access to pornography and other explicit imagery online means that it's much harder to protect children from "adult" images. According to a 2023 Common Sense Media report, 73 percent of teens ages thirteen to seventeen reported that they have seen online pornography. The average age kids first saw online pornography was twelve years old—with some 15 percent seeing it by age eleven or younger. About a third of those surveyed said they came upon it by accident, and nearly half said they were seeking it out. Boys are by and large more likely to seek out porn and report that it provides them with helpful information about sex.[12]

Even if you place careful restrictions on your own phones and computers, you can't guarantee that other families will do the same, and that your child won't be exposed to explicit content at a playdate or sleepover. Remember the days of finding a *Playboy* magazine? Most parents recall the shock and awe of opening up a magazine and seeing naked images. Engaging with porn has long been a part of how young people explore sexuality, but the problem is easy access to this kind of content can be harmful to a young child.

> Fortunately, research shows that when parents have conversations with their children about porn, this can help mitigate and protect young people from harm.[13]
>
> During middle childhood, you can keep the conversation pretty basic and straightforward—and this is probably a talk that's most appropriate for the nine to twelve age group. One way to start is by asking your child questions: "Do you ever hear other kids talking about something called porn?" or "Do you know what that is?" or "Have you ever seen it?" Reassure your child that they won't get into trouble if they tell you. Then say, "Here's what you need to know about porn: it is an adult movie that shows people without clothes on doing private things that are not real. It isn't what sex between people is really like. It's actors performing in a very over-the-top way. It's not meant for kids and is harmful for kids to watch. If you want to know about sex or what men and women's private parts look like, you can come to me, and I can help you learn in a way that's safe and real."

Looking Ahead

It's important to know that your child will very likely be curious about sex, and be prepared for the fact that they may be interested in seeking out porn to learn more. You will want to safeguard your child by setting up browser filters, activating parental controls on all devices, and looking into software and even hardware options. But ultimately, the more open you can be about talking about the things they may be curious about, the better you can protect them from viewing sexual content online.

Gender Identity

"Gender identity" refers to a person's internal sense of their own gender, which may or may not align with the sexual reproductive system with which they were born. This type of identity is *entirely separate* from sexual identity, something that often trips parents up, as they tend to conflate the two. Positive gender identity development means that a child is allowed to feel comfortable experiencing and expressing their sense of gender that's individual to them. I'm not just talking about trans and gender-nonconforming kids here. I'm talking about the entire spectrum of ways that your child might feel about their gender and how they express that. Your child might be a "girlie girl," obsessed with clothes and makeup, or she might be a "tomboy," only wearing jeans and T-shirts and wanting to climb trees. Your son might love to play with LEGOs and trucks, or he might prefer dolls and cooking.

The number one thing that you can do as a parent in order to foster positive gender identity development is to respect and affirm the way that your child expresses gender. If your son wants to cook, foster that. If your daughter wants to climb trees, foster that too. When you do this, you're encouraging the kind of internal acceptance and well-being your child can carry with them throughout life, so that they can feel acknowledged, accepted, and comfortable in expressing their gender identity authentically. The second most important thing you can do when your child is exploring their sense of gender is to be open with them. When parents value open communication, when they have an awareness of diverse gender identities, a child can ultimately flourish, even as they might initially struggle to figure out where they fit in. Over time, how a child is raised, what is reinforced, and what is avoided, will shape their identity formation and expression.

Although there aren't strict "stages" of gender identity development, I find it can be helpful for parents to understand that there are different phases, with kids going through a process of self-discovery and understanding over time. Experiences within this can differ, with some kids having a clear and consistent sense of their gender identity from an early age and with others experiencing shifts and exploration throughout their lives.

For your reference, here's a general overview of typical gender identity development.

INFANCY AND EARLY CHILDHOOD: AGES ZERO TO FIVE

In the earliest stages, children start to become aware of gender as a concept. They may observe differences in the ways boys and girls are treated, dressed, or expected to behave. However, their understanding of their own gender identity is still in the very early stages of formation. Specifically, between the ages of eighteen to twenty-four months a child starts to label others as boys or girls. By about the age of three years old they start to identify themself as a boy or girl. By four, they develop an even stronger sense of whether they identify as a boy or a girl. This period often involves gender exploration through play and social interactions. And at about four to five years old children have a solid sense of their gender identity.

MIDDLE CHILDHOOD: AGES SIX TO TWELVE

By middle childhood, children usually have a more formed sense of their gender identity. By now, they understand and identify with the gender they feel internally. During this time, societal expectations and cultural influences also play a role in shaping their understanding of gender roles.

ADOLESCENCE: AGES TWELVE TO EIGHTEEN

Adolescence is a *critical* period for gender identity development. Many teens become more settled on their own gender identity during this age and may question or explore their feelings around gender and attraction. For some, this may involve questioning societal norms and expectations related to gender. Now they're expressing it and finding friends who are as well.

Gender and Social Constructs

The reality is that we live in a culture where social constructs around gender—the ideas, values, stereotypes, and assumptions about gender such as "boys don't cry" and "girls are sugar and spice and everything nice"—are still rife. These constructs can help and hurt boys, girls, and gender-nonconforming kids alike.

In the world of psychology, there's no longer a debate about nature versus nurture in children—it is quite clear that both nature *and* nurture play a part in shaping the people kids become. And there do seem to be some qualities related to biological gender that are baked-in from birth. By and large, boys would rather play with trucks, cars, and balls; they are more active, do more roughhousing, and they prefer to play with other boys. This is believed to be because of their higher levels of prenatal testosterone in the womb.

The majority of little girls really do prefer dolls and pink dresses and are more likely to play quietly in groups, preferring imaginative play. This doesn't mean that there aren't children whose sense of gender expression falls outside of this binary; it's just that the majority are socialized to conform to these toys and play styles that are often unconsciously guided by parents and caregivers based on cultural expectations and their own experiences.

What happens as children grow older is that they get socialized in ways that reinforce these tendencies. During puberty boys get their next wave of testosterone, which tends to make them more interested in sex than their female counterparts. Girls, meanwhile, may begin wanting to wear makeup and dress in ways that are provocative. However, it's still the way children are raised and socialized by the parents and other adults around them that really shapes them. Harmful gendered stereotypes and sayings like "Boys will be boys" or "Girls are teases" reinforces that boys can treat girls any way they want and that girls are somehow to blame for attracting unwanted attention. This is why it's so important for parents, teachers, and coaches to model clear expectations for both boys and girls through doing things like offering a diverse variety of toys to play with, being open to various activities and sports, challenging stereotypes, and emphasizing the importance of inclusivity.

As a parent, it's a good idea to be mindful of all the ways the gender binary can hurt children. Let's look at some of these.

SOCIAL CONSTRUCTS FOR BOYS

Social constructs for boys dictate that a boy's personality should be strong, decisive, dominant, competitive, prideful, independent, fearless, aggressive, and adventurous. A boy tends to be more valued when he is tall, muscular, and strong.

How this hurts boys:

Thanks to these social constructs, boys can get the idea they always need to be tough and strong, so they tend to underreport sexual abuse or bullying. In general, society has a higher tolerance for violence and assault against boys (until 2012, the rape of adult males wasn't even legally acknowledged). As they get older and enter the teen years, boys may be less likely to ask for help when they need it because they've internalized the message that they need to be strong and independent. Boys may be less likely to explore interests that are outside of the masculine norm such as art, cooking, dance, or design for fear of rejection from peers. They may not feel as if they can play with dolls, or play house, which robs them of an opportunity to practice nurturance, gentleness, and compassion, as well as differing gender roles. Parents are less likely to talk to boys about how they feel, and they pay more attention to their emotions of anger rather than sadness. And the more screen time they have the more it gets reinforced that they are "the superior sex," which can perpetuate misogyny and sexism.

SOCIAL CONSTRUCTS FOR GIRLS

Girls are expected to be cooperative, relationship-focused, pleasers and peacemakers, poised and graceful. Their expected dominant emotions are sensitive, empathic, nurturing, dramatic, and emotional. Physically, more emphasis is placed on looks, clothes, and being "pretty" than it is for boys.

Girls get strong messages about the importance of what they wear or how they look, which means they're less likely to be encouraged to play rough or with trucks or dirt, and this robs them of the opportunity to practice assertiveness and a broader range of conflict-resolution skills. This may affect the range of careers that they assume are open to them in the future, if they don't feel like those roles are "for girls." They may get the idea that they should be nurturers, taking care of others, which may mean they grow up to neglect their own needs. Low self-esteem in girls and issues with body image can affect a girl's confidence and mental health.

WHAT YOU CAN DO TO MAKE SURE SOCIAL CONSTRUCTS DON'T LIMIT YOUR CHILD

- Seeing parents in a variety of roles gives children a chance to see the potential ways that their gender identity can be expressed. Are they into sports and cars like their dad? Do they enjoy baking like their mom? Maybe Dad's the one who's into cooking and Mom's into sports. Or maybe they have two moms, two dads, or a single mom or dad. As best you can, model gender equality with your child.

- Allow your child to have a full range of activities and toys. Don't limit them to "girls' activities" or "boys' activities."
- Expose them to media that offer them a range of role models: from men who sideline their careers to stay at home to raise children, to women who are bosses and travel for work.
- Research shows that at birth, both boys and girls are wired equally for relationship and connection. However, repeated studies have shown that baby girls are better with self-soothing (the beginning of self-regulation), and baby boys need more help to calm down. This seems to persist as children grow older—boys need more help calming down and learning to regulate their emotions from their parents. What can we do? Be mindful of how you treat your boys and how you support their feelings, and teach them to self-regulate.

Understanding Gender Expression

Prior to puberty, you may have still decided which clothes, shoes, and accessories your kid would wear. You may have bought these things without your child even being with you. You may have styled their hair in the morning and chosen which products to use on their bodies. At this age, gender expression begins to play a big part in how your child wants to present themselves to the world, and once puberty gets going, it is totally normal for a child to have their own ideas of what they want to wear, how they want to do their own hair, and which products they want to use. A child will begin to express their sense of gender through clothing, makeup, perfume or cologne, jewelry, shoes, hairstyles, and accessories—and this expression can become a strong part of a child's identity. You may not like your child's choices. You may not agree with their style as these new looks may or may not align with your expectations or the norms of your community. And because puberty starts earlier for some kids, these may be negotiations you didn't expect to be having at nine and ten years old. But I want to reassure you that this is all *entirely normal*.

I remember working with a family whose eleven-year-old daughter wanted to dress provocatively in short skirts and crop tops. The parents didn't know what to do. On the one hand, they didn't feel the way she dressed was appropriate. On the other hand, they didn't want to blame or shame her for her clothing choices. I counseled them that this was a good opportunity to teach their daughter a life lesson: that we have to wear clothing that's appropriate for different occasions, settings, and contexts. For example, they could tell their daughter that she could dress however she liked while hanging out with her friends at the mall, but when it came time to go to church on Sunday, or visit her grandparents, or go to school, or babysit, she needed to wear more modest attire. The same principle can be applied for boys who want to wear shorts in winter, or wear sweatpants and sneakers to a formal event. Teaching kids about context-dependent dressing is actually important and can help them as they grow up and begin to express themselves to the world.

Understanding Gender Nonconformity

I first met Skye when she went by a different name and used the pronouns, she/her. Skye was about ten years old in one of my puberty classes. In the two classes she attended, I could tell that she was uncomfortable in her own skin: she kept her eyes on the ground, rarely looked up at me, and didn't engage as readily as the other girls. After we'd finished, her mother asked me if I could meet with her individually for therapy as Skye was shut down and had no friends. I said sure, and Skye and I embarked on a journey of gender identity exploration that taught me so much about understanding and managing these issues in puberty.

Skye (now they/them) had grown up never feeling as if they were female, and so the earliest discussions we had together had to do with their name. At the time they were still going by their birth name, but over a period of sessions, Skye wanted to change their name to something that was gender neutral. They tried on different names over a period of time at school until they settled on Skye. As time went on, Skye began to tell their parents and extended family that they wanted to be known by this new name, and by and large, their relatives were supportive. In sixth grade, Skye decided they wanted to go by the pronouns they/them to reflect their nonbinary identity. Again, the family went through a period of transition where they got accustomed to the new pronouns. It wasn't always easy for Skye's parents, especially when it came to explaining to family and teachers, but they read the statistics around LGBTQ+ youth that clearly indicate that supporting your child is the best way to help safeguard against the kinds of mental health issues that typically affect this group of young people.

What Skye was going through was a period of gender identity exploration. From a psychological perspective, this is *a normal stage of child development*. Sexual development includes the exploration of gender identity. It's a process that involves a child understanding and defining whether they identify as the sex they were born—if they were born a boy, do they feel male? If they were born a girl, do they feel female? **I want to make clear that this is not some woke, modern model of child development.** This is the way it has always been—it's a part of puberty. And if you are thinking to yourself that you don't recall ever pondering whether you felt male or female, it likely indicates that you identified with your gender assigned at birth, that your sex and gender matched.

Every child, whether they are exploring a different gender identity from their biological one or not, goes through a period of figuring out who they are in middle childhood, and through the process they reveal more about who they are and who they want to become to those around them. This can take the form of deciding which friends they prefer, which activities they like to do, which shows they like to watch, who they have a crush on, or which gender they identify with—or don't. Identity at this age is not fixed, it's developing, and it has a lot to do with a child starting to understand where they fit in the world. On the most basic level, your role as a parent is to help your kid become comfortable with who they really are.

I know there will be readers coming to this topic with varying levels of discomfort, who wish we could "just go back to a time when we just had two genders, end of discussion." But the reality is that your child is growing up in a world where this is a part of life. My belief is that knowledge is power. If we are going to have strong opinions about an issue that affects a relatively small percentage of children (1 percent of the US population in 2021, according to the US Census Bureau[14]) we should be educated about it. Nonbinary and gender-nonconforming kids do exist, they always have, it's just that in the last decade they've become much more visible. It is true that this kind of identification—or at least the reporting of it—is on the rise, and so if it isn't your child who is exploring their gender identity, then there will be someone else's child in your community who is. My point of view is that if you don't feel comfortable with something—whether it's gender nonconformity or something else—the best thing you can do is to educate yourself. In the case of gender issues, getting educated doesn't have to mean you change your personal opinion, but it can mean that you can have conversations with your child that are more informed and empathic and help bridge gaps between different viewpoints.

Understanding Gender Dysphoria

Gender dysphoria occurs when there's a conflict between the sex you were assigned at birth and the gender with which you identify ("dysphoria" meaning when someone experiences a significant amount of distress, uneasiness, and dissatisfaction).[15] Studies reveal that by the age of seven, 73 percent of transgender women and 78 percent of transgender men will have experienced some kind of gender dysphoria, although not all people who identify as trans experience gender dysphoria. Being transgender is considered an identity, not a medical condition.

Although gender dysphoria can start to present in very early childhood, it usually intensifies as puberty hits, often causing serious distress and making a child feel extremely uncomfortable in their own body. I have had kids describe their gender dysphoria to me like "keeping a yearslong secret." Looking back at early childhood, they feel as if they were living a lie, but they didn't know what to do or who to go to.

This issue may seem new to parents who are wondering why they hadn't ever heard about or knew anyone with gender dysphoria when they were a child. Although the phenomenon may not have been part of the mainstream conversation back then, the reality is that for professionals in the fields of psychology, psychiatry, and medicine, this subject is actually not new at all. Psychologists have long been concerned with the issue of gender dysphoria because of the mental health issues that often accompany it, as well as increased risk factors that include substance abuse, self-harming behaviors, and suicide attempts. Beginning in the 1910s, the German physician Magnus Hirschfeld conducted groundbreaking research on individuals experiencing gender dysphoria. In the 1950s and 60s, pioneering physicians like David Cauldwell and Harry Benjamin came up with diagnostic terms related to gender identity and began publishing books on the subject. Only recently, a cache of letters surfaced, written to Benjamin in the 1960s from children as young as seven and eight who had heard about his work and wanted to share their experiences with him.

Looking Ahead

If you can have a better understanding of gender and sexual child development now—and if you can have open and supportive conversations with your six- to twelve-year-old child at this time—then you're going to be in a much better position to talk to them about these topics as they enter the teenage years. You will have laid a strong foundation, so that they will be much more likely to come to you for support when the stakes are so much higher and they're navigating a whole range of issues around romantic and sexual relationships, including safe sex, consent, and pregnancy prevention.

In a Nutshell

My hope is that this chapter has helped you not only to have a better understanding of sexuality and gender as they relate to normal child development, but that you feel more confident of what you can do to ensure your child remains mentally healthy as they grow and explore their sexual and gender identity. Here's a summary of the tips covered in this chapter:

- Talk to your child about sex, sexuality, and gender in an open, nonjudgmental, age-appropriate way. If you don't talk to them about these topics, they will likely learn from Google or their peers.
- Model consent for your child. When you set boundaries and expectations—and stick to them—you're showing them what consent looks like. At the same time, give your child autonomy over their body, allow them their privacy and a voice on issues like whether you post photos of them online.
- Talk to your child about pornography and monitor and restrict their online access.
- If your child comes to you and says they're attracted to someone of their own sex or the opposite sex—meet them where they are. Don't say, "You're too young." Say "Tell me more about that" and "It's okay to ask questions at this age—you're figuring things out."
- Teach your child to be open-minded and a good ally to their LGBTQ+ peers. These children are much more prone to mental health problems than their peers and need you and your child's support more than ever.
- If your child comes out to you as LGBTQ+, it's very important not to dismiss them or try to convince them to change. Instead, it's vital to support and validate them. This is the number one way to protect them from internalized stigma and mental health issues.
- Understand that exploring gender identity is a normal part of child development and accept your child for who they are, whether they conform to typical gender norms or not.

PART III

The Tough Stuff

CHAPTER 7

Body Image and Relationship with Food

> It is literally impossible to be a woman. You are so beautiful, and so smart, and it kills me that you don't think you're good enough. Like, we have to always be extraordinary, but somehow we're always doing it wrong. You have to be thin, but not too thin. And you can never say you want to be thin. You have to say you want to be healthy, but also you have to be thin . . .
>
> —Gloria played by America Ferrara, excerpt from the *Barbie* movie

This chapter explores topics related to body image and personal relationships with food, including discussions on eating disorders, diet culture, and body dysmorphia. Some readers may find the content emotionally triggering. If you are struggling with these issues, consider reaching out to a health care provider or counselor for support.

Although I've worked with many clients with body image issues over my years in practice, Leila, who was in sixth grade at the time we met, stands out. Her mom had initially contacted me about her daughter's anxiety and low self-esteem, but when eleven-year-old Leila arrived at our first session she explained that she had been doing her own research.

"I've been looking online," she told me. "I think I have body dysmorphic disorder."

That day at my clinic, I completed an evaluation, and sure enough, Leila seemed to be right. Body dysmorphic disorder (BDD) is when a person has an intense and overwhelming fixation on aspects of their body that they want to change. For Leila, this meant checking herself in the mirror dozens of times a day, excessively looking at her face, constantly picking at the acne on her skin, along with an irrational belief that her nose was too big leading her to constantly take pictures of herself in profile. At school and home, Leila would joke about her body fixations, poking fun at herself, and so at first, her parents had been able to brush off some of these behaviors as a "phase." But by the time her parents brought her to me, she was skipping meals and only eating a small amount of the food on her plate. They were rightly concerned.

This disorder, which is a type of obsessive-compulsive disorder (OCD), hadn't arrived out of nowhere for Leila. When she was younger, her parents told me, she'd shown signs of OCD: she had to do things according to certain patterns, for example if she missed a step in her getting dressed routine, she had to start all over again. At the time, her parents just assumed she was somewhat anxious and that she would grow out of it. The problem was that now that Leila was in middle school, her fixations had intensified—and all those trips to the bathroom had disrupted her learning. When she went on vacation, she didn't want to be in a bathing suit because she thought she was "fat" (though she was below average weight for her height and age). Leila was a dancer and I learned that, like most of the other girls on the team, she had begun fixating on her abs, but in her case, it had become what we call a preoccupation.

After my initial assessment, I met with her parents to review my impressions and recommendations. They were worried, confused, and unsure of what to say or do. "We don't understand," they told me. "She's so beautiful, smart, and kind. Everyone loves her. She's only eleven. Why is this happening?" I told them that I understood how they were feeling and that I see parents every week who are blindsided that elementary and middle school–age children can feel this way. I reassured Leila's parents that they had done the right thing by intervening before Leila's obsessions had become a larger problem. "This isn't a phase that she will likely just grow out of," I told them. "This is different. These obsessions tend to build on themselves and get worse."

Leila and I worked together throughout the middle school years to help lessen the hold body dysmorphia had on her life. I brought onboard a nutritionist who specialized in disordered eating. When we started working together, Leila only wanted to eat at home; she would never eat out. If friends wanted to walk to get fast food after school, she would become extremely distressed and have to make up excuses not to go, bursting into tears at home because she was missing out on time with friends. The nutritionist created a spreadsheet for Leila that included all kinds of food, *including* fast food. When her friends wanted to go get a burger, we encouraged Leila to go with them. The first couple of times she went, she didn't eat anything. The next time she got a drink. Then the time after that she was able to order some fries, even if she didn't finish them. And we built up from there, until she could manage an actual burger. This was the slow, incremental work of what's known as "exposure and response prevention," gradually introducing someone to the very thing they are avoiding.

I also asked Leila to download a mental health app that she could use for journaling and tracking her triggers, her mirror checking, and her negative thinking about her body. She began to keep a log of the number of times she checked her body in the mirror every day, which is how we learned she was doing this as many as one hundred times a day. Leila was also having intrusive thoughts—uninvited, negative thinking. After tracking these thoughts in the app, we learned, with the exception of about three hours a day, she was constantly having negative thoughts about herself, convinced that people must be staring at her because her nose was so "big," her laugh was so "stupid," her thighs were so "fat." As hard as it was for Leila to track every single thought, it was actually really helpful for her to tally them in this way. She told me, "I knew it was happening a lot, but I didn't know it was this much."

Together, we worked on what are called replacement behaviors. Instead of checking herself multiple times in the full-length mirror, Leila was allowed to check herself once in the morning when she was fully dressed and only in the bathroom mirror (waist up). When she had the compulsion to look in the mirror at school, she had to go to the bathroom with the smaller mirror, and only three times a day. Leila was motivated and honest: as we worked on reducing the number of times she checked mirrors, she confessed to me that she had started checking her reflection in glass doors and windows instead. We slowly worked on getting her to just look at her reflection once and then keep walking.

We got her parents involved too. Their job was to monitor Leila's eating, to make sure that she had breakfast and dinner as she didn't eat lunch at school. Breakfast was hard for Leila but dinner she didn't have any trouble with—probably because she was hungry due to skipping lunch. Her parents modified the way they spoke to her about their own bodies, no longer making comments about "needing to lose weight for a vacation" or "skipping the dessert because it's fattening." I told her parents that I believed bringing their daughter in for treatment had prevented a full-blown eating disorder (ED).

Sadly, Leila's struggles with body image are not uncommon. Almost every week in my practice, I get an inquiry that reads something like this:

"I'm reaching out to you today because my ten-year-old daughter seems depressed. She has been saying things about being too fat and wanting to go on a diet. She's asked me what it means to count calories and asked if I thought it would help her if she learned how to do that."

"My nine-year-old son is saying that he doesn't want to eat fast food anymore and wants me to cook healthier. He doesn't want to eat school lunches. He said 'no' the other day at a birthday party to a slice of pizza and seems obsessed with everything he eats. When his dad and I ask him why, he says that those foods are unhealthy and gross and aren't good for him. We can't really disagree, but he seems to be taking this to an extreme."

It's crucial for parents to recognize that puberty represents a significant period of vulnerability for children, particularly concerning body image issues, and especially—but not exclusively—among girls. To add to this pressure, our children are being inundated with visuals on social media of thin, filter-enhanced tweens, teens, and young women wearing all kinds of makeup, sporting workout outfits, and promoting beauty products. They're being exposed to toxic beauty culture and figuring out how they fit within that—and as a result, they can be extremely self-conscious of their own perceived defects.

In my practice, it's rare to encounter a tween girl who doesn't have at least one negative thought about her appearance. These girls want to be skinny, but not too skinny; they want to have muscular legs, but not too big; they want to wear makeup to hide blemishes but look natural at the same time; and they want to have highlighted, sleek, straight hair, or the perfect beach-wave curl; I see girls as young as ten who follow along with "Get Ready with Me" routines, complete with cute outfits usually comprising cropped tops and leggings. These girls are captivated by beauty products, often displaying a preference for particular brands, with a tendency toward the most expensive ones at Sephora or in a TikTok Shop.

Many parents assume that body image problems are a high school issue affecting girls only. In fact, this is happening to kids at younger ages, and although girls are most likely to be susceptible, it's important to be aware that boys can become fixated on physical flaws, too. A 2015 report found that one-third of boys aged six to eight want thinner bodies. This same report also found more than half of girls want to be skinnier and that the average age for a girl to begin dieting is age eight. Eight![1]

An earlier study showed that nearly a third of children aged five to six chose an ideal body size that was thinner than their current perceived size. In fact, it has been reported that children as young as three years old worry about being "fat."[2] By age six, children are aware of dieting, and by the time they are seven years old, one in four children has engaged in some kind of dieting behavior.[3] Clearly, this is not an issue that kicks in when children are in high school—it's absolutely an elementary and middle school issue.

The question facing parents is when and how to intervene if you see concerning signs. As I explained to Leila's parents, having a poor body image can lead to disordered eating or an actual ED down the line if ignored. And puberty is a risk factor for children and EDs, because it's a period when kids gain a greater awareness of their bodies and the changes going on and may struggle with feelings of shame or ambivalence about growing up, paired with decreased self-esteem and comparison to peers. The further along a child is into puberty or the earlier the timing of the start of puberty increases these risks, particularly in girls.[4]

Body image and mental health are interrelated and complicated, and the stakes are high: there can be serious potential consequences if a child doesn't develop healthy self-esteem around her body. My goal here is to help walk you through how a child's sense of body image develops in middle childhood (a normal developmental process), while also laying out the warning signs for poor body image and disordered eating. We know increasing numbers of younger girls and boys are being affected, and that early intervention is essential for minimizing harm. So, my message to you is: don't wait until your child is older to begin guiding her on these issues. Now's the time.

Sound Familiar?

- Your child is talking about wanting to look a different way, being skinnier or more muscular and comparing herself to others. Telling her she's beautiful the way she is doesn't seem to be helping.
- Your child is already talking about avoiding certain foods because they're not good for her, and you're not sure what to say or how to respond.
- Your child is now competing in sports, and you notice that she's working out a lot, doing sit-ups late at night, and staring in the mirror frequently. You can't tell if this is a problem or helpful for her sport.
- You notice that your child is self-conscious about her weight and/or changing body—yet her body type clearly runs in your family, and you don't know if you should say something, especially since she hasn't said anything to you about it.
- Your child is all of a sudden not eating as much, shuffling food around her plate, and skipping meals. When you ask her about it, she says she's just not hungry. You don't want to make too big of a deal about it, but you're not sure when you should be concerned.
- You notice your child has gained weight in the past year and you don't know if this is normal or if you should be concerned—and you don't want to say anything to make your child feel uncomfortable or self-conscious.
- Your child comes home and tells you that some kids at school made a comment about her being "fat." You also don't know what to say to comfort her or guide her as to how she should handle it.

PARADIGM SHIFT

Paradigm: Negative body image and disordered eating is something that affects teenage girls. Younger girls and boys in general don't yet have to deal with this.

> **Shift:** Negative body image and disordered eating—as well as obesity—are on the rise and affecting younger kids, and not just girls but boys as well. Parents need to learn the signs in both girls and boys so they can respond and support them, and to prevent these issues from becoming serious problems as they grow older.

Why We All Need to Stop Commenting on Children's Bodies

Put yourself in the shoes of an eleven-year-old girl who's just gone through a growth spurt. Everywhere she goes, multiple times a week, people tell her, "Oh, you've gotten so tall!" or "I can't believe how grown-up you look!" or "Look at you, you're a young woman now!" Although these comments are well-meaning, the child on the other end of these "compliments" may not receive them that way. After all, her growth spurt isn't something she worked hard to attain, or that she feels she's earned, it's just something that happened to her. When you tell a kid, "You've gotten so tall!" she may smile awkwardly, but after that there's really nowhere else for the conversation to go, plus, you've inadvertently sent her the message that she's being judged on her appearance before anything else.

The next time you run into a child you haven't seen in a while who's suddenly grown or changed in some way, remember, you could be the fifth person to comment on her body that day. Instead of commenting on her looks, try asking her a question about her ("Are you still going to camp this summer?" "What are you learning in math class these days?") or sharing a memory of the last time you saw her. You don't need to reinforce or objectify society's obsession with looks to show your happiness to see her.

If you are wondering how you *can* compliment a child about the way she looks, I would encourage you to think about using your words to highlight a quality or characteristic that is actually within that child's control, rather than something due to genetics and outside of her control. This may sound like "I love your outfit. You have such a cool style!" or "I love the way you braided your hair. It shows off your highlights and how long it's getting!"

Body Image Issues: A Primer

When your child looks in the mirror, does she like what she sees? Whether the answer is yes, no, or sometimes can impact both her mental and physical health, including how active or involved in sports she is, all the way to being an indicator of her risk for an ED.

Body image development begins in early childhood. Very young children begin to develop a sense of body image around age four, alongside their physical, cognitive, and social growth. This sense of body image is wholly subjective: it's about how *she* thinks and feels about her own body. As a child grows and moves into middle childhood, she will also begin to take into account how she imagines *others* perceive her body. In this way, body image becomes an aspect of her identity. Kids tend to self-identify by the different groups they belong to—a soccer player, a Girl Scout, a musician, an artist. Body image is one aspect of a person's complete identity, and within it a child can hold different beliefs, even ones that contradict one another.

Body image exists on a continuum. On one end of the body image continuum, there's a positive body image, and on the other end there's a negative body image. The middle is composed of varying degrees of many different images—which is where most kids are. Body image can vary over time, with children feeling different ways about their bodies during different stages of their lives. Many factors contribute to a child's body image, including genetics, the environment she grows up in, her socioeconomic background, religious affiliation, and of course, the media she's exposed to.

Media influence is of particular importance in young children's lives, with social media, advertising, pop culture, and unrealistic beauty standards having a huge impact on a child's sense of herself. A series of Stanford University School of Medicine studies conducted on the island of Fiji before and after Western TV was brought to the country shows just how impactful media can be.[5] Prior to the arrival of Western TV, there were no known cases of EDs in

Fiji—but after it was introduced, body image and problematic eating behaviors started being reported, with higher rates of disordered eating such as restrictive dieting and purging.

Media plays a big role, but a child's personal history and upbringing can also impact the way she perceives herself and her body. For example, if a child is raised in a household or social environment in which a person's value is very closely tied to physical appearance, that child may begin to perceive her body as a measure of her self-worth. Conversely, if a child is raised in a home where parents express positive attitudes toward their own bodies, and avoid making negative comments about their appearance, children are more likely to adopt similarly positive attitudes.

The Self-Esteem Connection

As a parent, it's important to understand that there's a direct correlation between self-esteem and body image. I describe it this way to kids in my practice: self-esteem is liking yourself; it's when you feel worthy of taking up space and time; it's when you believe in yourself and know what you can do well. It also means knowing what you *aren't* so great at and being okay with that. By the age of five, children have self-esteem "comparable in strength to that of adults," according to a University of Washington study.[6] One of the more favorable outcomes of having positive self-esteem is that you have the confidence to try new things.

When kids are confident and secure about who they are, they're more likely to have a growth mindset. That means they can motivate themselves to take on new challenges and cope with and learn from mistakes. They're also more likely to stand up for themselves and ask for help when they need it. Research shows that kids with healthier self-esteem are more resilient and can feel proud even when they make a mistake. They are more independent and have a greater internal locus of control, which means they feel responsible for their own actions and decisions. Socially, they have healthier relationships with others, and have an easier time resisting peer pressure. They're also less likely to base their entire self-worth on their appearance, and more likely to validate themselves in other ways.

As if that weren't promising enough: positive self-esteem can act as a buffer against negative body image, helping kids maintain a more balanced perspective regarding their physical appearance. A child with a strong sense of self-esteem is more likely to appreciate her body for its functionality and overall health—what it can actually do—rather than conforming to high or unrealistic standards of beauty.

However, if your child doesn't have positive self-esteem yet, she's not alone. In fact, according to a paper published in the journal *Psychological Bulletin*, the greatest increase in self-esteem occurs during childhood and adulthood; notably, adolescence is not typically a time of increased self-esteem. The middle childhood years are an opportunity to build them up before the dips in the teen years. During middle childhood, as she develops socially and cognitively, and gains some independence and mastery, self-esteem develops alongside this process, with levels then seeming to plateau in early to middle adolescence (ages eleven to fifteen).[7]

Here's what you can do to help build up your child's self-esteem in general:

- When a child knows that she's valued for the person she *is*, not just what she does, this contributes to a positive self-image. Embrace and celebrate your child's uniqueness. Encourage her to express herself and pursue activities that align with her passions. Allow her to take reasonable risks and expect some failure. Don't remove all obstacles out of her way—she needs to overcome some adversity to build up a sense of self-worth and confidence.
- Make sure to give your child positive reinforcement for attributes beyond appearance, such as intelligence and kindness. The things that children are praised for or complimented on in childhood can have long-lasting effects. I bet you can still recall something positive (or negative) someone once told you when you were a child that has stayed with you to this day. I remember being told I was a good writer by an English teacher in junior high, and that's stuck with me all these years. It's always tempting to compliment your child on her appearance (particularly when you're the parent and naturally adore the way she looks) but make sure to balance those compliments with observations about the things she does and who she is.
- Be judicious in your praise; don't praise every little thing your child does. When you do praise your child, make sure you do so in a way that

teaches her to be proud of her efforts and accomplishments. Focus on the process she went through to achieve something rather than just the outcome. Instead of saying, "Great job, you got an A in your school project!" You can say, "I'm so proud of how hard you worked on that project, staying after school, leading your group, and learning about the topic. And even more importantly, you should be too!" Acknowledge and celebrate what she's been doing and the improvements that she's made along the way, not just the end result. This reinforces the idea that learning, and growth are ongoing processes and it's the effort that counts.

- Model positive self-talk and a healthy self-image for your child. Children learn best by observing their parents, so when you model a positive attitude toward yourself, this can be a really good way to get your child to do the same. If your child hears you expressing positive attitudes toward your work, your life, and your body, there's a much greater likelihood that your child will talk and think positively about herself too. Children who can talk to themselves positively have a much better time when facing a challenge and attempting to problem-solve.
- Encourage friendships. How kids relate to one another is a big part of building self-esteem. Interacting positively with peers fosters a sense of belonging and contributes to feelings of self-worth. Just having one friend who listens, "gets" you, and accepts you for who you are can make all the difference.
- Encourage your child to develop talents and skills. Emphasizing and encouraging a child's talents, skills, and interests helps her develop a strong sense of self-esteem that goes far beyond physical appearance.
- Teach your child to have self-compassion. This involves emphasizing to your child that everyone is unique and has their own strengths and areas for growth.

Body Image Issues

Between the ages of six to twelve, children are thinking about their appearance and how they are seen by others. During the later years of middle childhood especially, appearance can become vital to self-esteem, as kids are judged on how they look more than at any other stage of their lives, with adults frequently commenting on their growth and newfound physical maturity. As a child becomes more physically developed, she'll likely begin comparing herself to peers. If a child perceives that her body is different from those around her—and if she feels she isn't being accepted socially as a result—this often causes doubts about her attractiveness, which can lead to overall low self-worth. She may feel bad about her body, but also her hair, her voice, her eye color, even her personality. When a child is consumed by these thoughts—whether she feels she's too fat, too skinny, too tall, or too short—it can become more difficult for her to pursue goals or new interests, and it can have a real effect on social connections, confidence, involvement in sports and activities, and more. The relationship between self-esteem and body image can then form a feedback loop with negative body image contributing to lower self-esteem, and lower self-esteem, in turn, exacerbating negative body image.

Just because your child isn't thrilled about some aspect of her body isn't necessarily cause for alarm. What would be a cause for concern is the way in which that sense of body image impacts her thoughts, feelings, and functioning. Remember, having body image *issues* is not a clinical diagnosis; it is a "condition" to pay attention to as it is a significant risk factor for EDs and other mental health issues.

Here are some red flags:

- Your child may tug on her shirts, want to wear things that are oversized or platform shoes to try to seem taller, or express that she wishes she was skinnier/more muscular.
- Your child may start to become more restrictive about what she eats, talking about cutting out certain foods and not wanting to finish the food on her plate.
- Your child may start to exercise excessively, often in her room at night, doing sit-ups and push-ups before she goes to bed. This type of excessive exercise is usually done independently and at night to burn off calories, part of a rigid routine that becomes ritualistic.
- You may hear your child talking about body image concerns or comparing herself to others.

- Your child may not want to wear a bathing suit at the beach or swimming pool because she's not comfortable with her body.
- Your child may begin avoiding certain other activities or opportunities such as going on a sleepover or a vacation because she doesn't feel comfortable in her body.

If you see any of these behaviors, you should start by having a conversation with your child. Instead of asking "What's going on?" you can begin with "I notice that. . . ." For example, if your child has been exercising excessively, you can say, "I notice you've been working out at night . . ." Remember to be gentle, nonjudgmental, and stick to open-ended questions like "I wonder why you started exercising like that all of a sudden?" In this way you might learn that your child is on a sports team with a kid who has abs, and she wants them too. You might learn that someone at her school told her she had a "fat tummy."

If your child tells you about these things, this is your chance to talk about healthy body image with her. Remember to emphasize that everybody's body is different and that it's being healthy that matters: "Your body is strong and healthy, it can run really fast, it can lift heavy things." You can also explain about the role of genetics, that "in our family we are tall, big-boned people," or "in our family we all have small frames and tend to be shorter than most people." I like to draw parallels between the diversity in body shapes and sizes and the variety of flowers in a garden. Just as we appreciate the unique beauty of roses, tulips, and sunflowers without expecting them to resemble each other, we should celebrate the individuality of our bodies. Just as each flower is created to bloom in its own way, so too are we uniquely formed and beautiful in our own ways.

Body Shaming

What It Is and How to Respond to It

Body shaming is a term that your child will likely have heard online or on the playground. It's a form of bullying[8] and it's what happens when someone says something inappropriate or derogatory about someone else's body size or shape. This might be in the form of "fat jokes," comments about how skinny someone looks, questions about what someone is wearing ("Do you think leggings look good on you?"), or when someone compares another person to an animal. These are the most obvious forms of body shaming, but there's also the kind of body shaming that can happen internally, when a kid says to herself, "I have big ears," or "I hate my legs," or "I'm the ugliest kid in the class."

Just like other forms of bullying, body shaming can have a negative impact on a child—and in this case it can even be a risk factor for BDD, so the best way to combat it is to address it. If you learn your child has been a victim of body shaming, you can say, "I'm so sorry you've had to experience that. It's not okay for anyone to make hurtful comments about your body or how you look, and I want you to know that I love and value you just the way you are. I understand why you feel upset about what happened, and I'm here to listen if you want to talk about it."

If at this point, your child seems engaged and wanting to keep talking, you can go on to say . . . "I know it can be hard to remember when you're feeling hurt, but people's unkind words say more about them than they do about you. What truly matters is how you feel about yourself." *Now . . . pause. Hold space. Try to read how she is feeling. Maybe hug her. Maybe hold or break eye contact. Stay attuned. Check in with yourself too: how are you feeling right now? Are you triggered? Breathe: it's okay if she can hear your long, deep breaths. You are regulating; she may need you to lead the breathing, she may be holding her breath to hold her feelings in.* Then say, "You're brave, kind, and beautiful inside and out, and I'm so sorry if anyone is making you doubt that in yourself."

If the body shaming is being done to another child who your child knows, you can encourage your child to stand up for them, and to tell the bully, "Don't say that—that's not kind and it's not true!" or ask an adult for help. You can also teach your child that it helps to then ask the child who's being mistreated to come with her or sit with that friend at lunch or recess for that extra support.

If your child is saying negative things to herself about her body, you can work with her on replacing those negative thoughts with positive ones. It can be helpful to have a simple sentence that she can say to herself when the negative thought comes up, something like "I am learning to love and accept myself just as I am."

On the other hand, if you discover that your child is body shaming another child, it's important to address this promptly and sensitively to teach her about respect for *every body* and use it as an opportunity to practice empathy. Start by addressing the situation in a straightforward and calm way. You can start by explaining to your child what body shaming is. You will want to provide her with specific examples of what you heard her say (if you know what was said or done). Make it clear that "saying these things is unacceptable because it's emotionally hurtful to others, even if the person goes along with it as a joke or smiles and laughs." I had a child once tell me that there was a group of boys in her class that were calling her younger sister a giraffe because she was the tallest girl in the class. She told me that the boys thought it was funny and her sister would just roll her eyes or ignore them at school, but that once she was home, she was tearful while telling her parents about what they were saying. Helping your child understand how their words or actions might make the other person feel is a lifelong skill that takes a lot of practice.

Ask questions like "How would you feel if someone said something similar about your body?" or "Can you imagine how the sister felt when this happened to her?" This can help her develop empathy and consider the impact of her actions on others. Emphasize that everyone's body is unique, like the flower garden we talked about earlier, and that it's important to respect others regardless of how they look on the outside. Finally, make sure your child understands that body shaming is never okay, and let them know the consequences of repeating this behavior like apologizing, losing privileges, or having to write a letter about why you don't treat people that way.

Body Dysmorphic Disorder (BDD)

As discussed, BDD is a severe form of poor body image that is closely connected to OCD.[9] This is a clinical diagnosis and a serious condition where a child may start to obsess about her appearance, becoming overly critical of perceived minor flaws, not just in her body but in her face and her appearance generally, as was the case with my client Leila. This condition goes above and beyond just not liking a certain physical trait or even poor body image, but really starts to become all-consuming, potentially leading to social isolation. BDD presents a heartbreaking challenge for families, as parents struggle to witness their child, whom they see as beautiful, consumed by fixation on perceived physical flaws.

Although the mean age of BDD diagnosis is sixteen, the average age of symptom onset is twelve, and it appears to affect girls at higher rates than boys in adolescence. In adulthood, rates among women and men eventually even out.[10] What seems to be clear is that there's a strong association between BDD and ED. Twenty-five years ago, BDD was nearly unheard of; today, it's thought to affect nearly 2.5 percent of adolescents and it's arguably one of the most impairing and high-risk mental health conditions. Negative thoughts about body image can consume a majority of a child's waking hours, becoming so distressing that she may experience anxiety or depression, or contemplate self-harm or even suicide.[11] Despite the serious nature of BDD, it's thought to be overlooked and not well understood.[12]

There's a lot we don't know about the exact causes of BDD. The disorder may be partly inherited as it tends to run in families. It may be caused by a low supply of serotonin, a chemical in the brain that's linked to mood and energy. And it may be due to brain differences as some areas of the brain look and work differently in people with BDD. It's important to remember that this disorder isn't due to anything a parent did or said.

When a child is affected by this condition, it can take a while to arrive at a diagnosis. Families will often visit dermatologists, aestheticians, and even plastic surgeons before they see a mental health practitioner. What starts out with treating acne can escalate to include coloring hair, buying expensive makeup, and eventually, a child who's asking for nose jobs, lip injections, and lash extensions. And many parents go along with this because they genuinely believe it will help the child. When families finally come in to see a psychologist like me, the reason for referral is rarely "body dysmorphia." Instead, the parent will usually say that the child has "poor self-esteem, difficulty with relationships, and isn't performing well in school." Many parents simply aren't aware of BDD, so it's important to know the signs as early detection and treatment are important.[13]

Here are some red flags that your child may be beginning to suffer from BDD:

- Your child may begin displaying repetitive behaviors such as mirror checking or repeatedly seeking validation or reassurance from others about her looks, hair, outfit, or perceived flaws. This may become compulsive and interfere with daily functioning and socializing as your child tries to manage her distress and anxiety about her body.
- Your child may brush her hair all the time and want to constantly change outfits.
- Your child may begin to be preoccupied with her appearance and excessively compare her appearance to others.
- Your child may begin picking at her skin.
- Your child may want to go to a dermatologist to get treated for acne, she may want to color her hair or have her teeth whitened, she may start using a lot of makeup or want to have other modifications to the way she looks.
- Your child may seem withdrawn, she may begin avoiding social situations or start to become isolated.
- Your child seems to be more distressed and anxious about her looks and appearance than in the past.
- Your child may become depressed, contemplate self-harm, or express suicidal thoughts.
- Your child may start to talk about wanting plastic surgery.
- Your child may start to have extreme exercise habits, which usually occur at night after dinner in order to burn off calories. You may find her doing sit-ups, jumping rope, or running in place.
- Your child may be feeling hopeless—she may realize that her perception of her body has somehow become warped, but she may assume that she has no way out of this. People with BDD often have a lot of shame around how they feel about their appearance and the thoughts that consume them.

If you see any more than two of these behaviors in your child, then you need to broach a conversation about this. Studies show that if children are directly asked about body image, they are much more likely to disclose their issues around it than if no one ever brings it up. You can begin gently with "I've noticed that you've been talking a lot about not liking your nose and wanting to buy more makeup—tell me about that . . ." In response, your child might say, "I think I'm ugly." This is the time where you're going to be very tempted to say, "But you're so beautiful!" The problem is, correcting a child in this way does not help her; it may even make her feel invalidated and ashamed that she doesn't see herself the way you do.

Pay attention to your own body's internal state while you have this conversation. You may be triggered by your child disclosing that she hates some aspect of her body or appearance. Checking in with yourself (your heartbeat, your stomach, your thoughts) first before you continue on will be helpful to the conversation. When you do this, you are practicing what are called interoceptive skills, which give you the ability to perceive and interpret bodily sensations, such as heartbeat, respiration, digestion, and emotional arousal. Interoceptive skills play a crucial role in various aspects of physical and mental health, including emotional regulation, stress management, and self-awareness. People with strong interoceptive skills are better able to recognize and understand their emotions, sensations, and needs, which can lead to greater awareness and better coping strategies.

Instead of trying to convince your child that there isn't anything wrong with her, you can take a deep breath and say, "How much are you thinking about this? Is it just every now and again or all the time?" If it's occasionally, that's okay, but if your child is thinking about how "ugly" she is all day long, that's concerning. Don't discount what your child is telling you, don't invalidate her, and do seek professional help if you feel you need it.

What Parents Can Do to Support a Positive Sense of Body Image

Parents have a tremendous influence over a child's sense of body image. Here are some ways to instill a positive image in your child:

- Make a habit of checking in with your child. Establishing an open line of communication allows children to express their feelings and concerns about their bodies without fear of judgment. If body development is a taboo topic in your home, and you never talk about it, your child may get the idea she can't come to you if/when issues arise. If your child *does* say that she doesn't like how she looks or wishes she could lose weight, don't ignore or overreact to what she's telling you. Calmly ask your child to tell you more so you can figure out her potential level of distress.
- Practice emotional check-ins for yourself—and your child. As a parent, it's important to practice regular emotional check-ins of your own when these topics come up. This might involve taking a few moments throughout the day to pause, breathe deeply, and tune in to your emotional state. You can ask yourself questions like:
  - *"How am I feeling right now?"*
  - *"What emotions am I experiencing?"*
  - *"Where do I feel these emotions in my body?"* (Practicing interoception skills: see above.)

  Encourage your child to do the same.
- Connect the dots between food and feelings. How we feel about our weight and whether we're compelled to go on a diet is closely intertwined with our mental health. Ask your child if she is feeling sad, does she lose her appetite? When she is feeling stressed, does she notice a change in her hunger cues? Food and feelings are connected with hunger and satiety, with people either consuming excess food or losing their appetite when strong emotions come up. Kids can excessively snack when anxious or stressed and they may find they don't feel like eating when they're depressed. The food and feelings connection is something your child should understand, but make sure to teach this in a nonjudgmental way. You can say, "Honey, I notice when you're stressed about a game you crave sweet foods . . ." or "When you feel left out you don't seem to want to eat dinner."
- Understand that what kids wear at this age is part of self-expression. Some children care a lot about what they wear, with fashion being a way for them to express their identity. If this is your child, remember to avoid complimenting her on how the clothing looks on her body and instead put the focus on her style, *how* she puts clothes together, and the way she's wearing them. Instead of saying, "You look so cute in that dress!" you can

say, "I love how you put your whole outfit together with the hairband and the purse!"
- Teach your child about media literacy. It's important to educate your child about the way bodies are presented in the media and help her develop critical thinking skills. You can explain to your child that images in the media are often edited or put through a filter and don't represent realistic body types. Make this an ongoing and regular conversation. Some schools teach media literacy or digital citizenship, but many don't, so it's really up to parents to take the lead here.
- Limit your child's exposure to unrealistic body standards. Yes, it is hard when unrealistic body standards are all around us, but when you control a child's exposure by monitoring her media content, you can really make a difference in how she perceives herself. No, you can't control everything—but even if you could cut her exposure by half, that would help.
- Allow your child to play with all kinds of toys, not just those dolls and action figures with extreme body shapes. I'm not saying banish Barbie and G.I. Joe from the toy box, but I am saying that you should give your child other options and make sure she understands that certain toys do not have realistic body shapes.
- Challenge gender stereotypes. When it comes to body image, it's a really good idea to challenge traditional gender norms and stereotypes. Explain to your child that boys don't have to be tall and muscular, and girls don't have to be petite and skinny. Then encourage your child to embrace her authentic self, regardless of societal expectations.
- Provide equal support. Both girls and boys may face body image challenges, so parents should be mindful of providing equal support and encouragement to all children, not just the girls. Don't discount your son's concerns about his body, even if you feel they're silly or not a big deal. If he starts asking, "When can I get braces?" it's possible he's feeling insecure about his teeth. When a boy wants a certain haircut, this means his hair is part of how he views himself, his self-expression. If he starts working out, it may mean he's self-conscious about his soft belly or his skinny arms. Validate him in the same way you would with a girl and be sensitive to his need to look a certain way, while staying on alert for warning signs that may mean he's becoming overly obsessive in his attention to his looks.

- Be a positive role model for your child. The reality is that significant numbers of adults have an unhealthy relationship with their bodies and/or food and so once you have children, if you haven't addressed your own issues yet, now is the time to be more mindful about them. Challenge yourself to address your attitude to your body and to model different ways of thinking of and relating to it. Many studies report a connection between a parent's attitude toward dieting and children's restrictive eating—in fact, studies show that a majority of girls as young as five years old will hold similar beliefs about dieting as their mothers.[14] If you're finding it really difficult to model healthy attitudes and behaviors around food and body image, you may need to seek out professional help for yourself.

Disordered Eating Behavior (DEB)

Keiran was twelve and in seventh grade when his parents first brought him to see me. They'd noticed that their son was bringing home most of the lunch they had packed for him. At dinner he would only eat grilled chicken, a salad, or vegetables, no rice or potatoes, except for once a week, and even though he eventually shared he was typically still hungry, he wouldn't allow himself to eat seconds of chicken. At night, he would sneak into the pantry and eat nuts, dried fruit, and if there were hard-boiled eggs in the refrigerator, he would take a few to his room. Once he was finished eating, he would do push-ups and sit-ups until he felt he burned off the calories. He shared with his parents that he had purged food at night the day of his twelfth birthday because he had "eaten bad" that day. He told them that this was the first and only time he did this.

By the time I met with Keiran he had been engaged in this eating cycle for about six months. He told me he had begun restricting his diet after starting cross-country running and noticing how slim the other boys' bodies were. He said he noticed that the best runners were all thin yet muscular and seemed to only eat protein, so slowly over the course of the fall and winter he started thinking about it a lot, and eventually started creating a habit that he said made him feel better at first. Eventually, he became obsessed and felt out of control. He told me that half his brain thought it was wrong and the other half thought he had it under control, that it wasn't really that bad.

As I explained to Keiran's parents, their son was displaying signs of disordered eating behaviors (DEB).

"Wait, disordered eating?" Keiran's father asked. "Does that mean that he has an eating disorder?"

I explained that DEB is *not* the same thing as an ED. Instead, disordered eating refers to a wide range of abnormal eating behaviors and attitudes toward food, weight, and body image that may not meet the criteria for an eating disorder but can still have a negative impact on a child's physical and emotional well-being. DEB is less severe in that it may not affect a child's ability to function in their everyday activities. Keiran was still going to school every day; he was attending regular activities. He didn't meet the criteria for an ED, but at the same time, he was definitely displaying signs of abnormal eating patterns, which is a risk factor for EDs.

Although most parents have heard of EDs such as anorexia and bulimia nervosa, few have an understanding of DEB. Yet this is something that you need to be aware of. Research has shown that children *younger than adolescents* may engage in DEB, according to the National Institute of Mental Health (NIMH).[15] A 2022 University of California, San Diego study published in *JAMA* revealed that DEB were found in 5 percent of nine- and ten-year-old children. This study also found that boys and girls were equally affected by DEB and that the higher the BMI, the more likely they were to develop DEB. Kids who started puberty earlier had a higher risk of DEB, and when kids are going through growth spurts, as they do at this age, they are more likely to be susceptible to DEB too.

DEB frequently involves many of the same behaviors that occur in EDs, such as a loss of appetite, eating for comfort, restricting certain foods, eating smaller portions, or occasionally binging and purging, but the symptoms occur less often (maybe once or twice a month) and/or less intensely (your child might not have an extreme fear of gaining weight, it's just that she doesn't want to gain any more weight). Although the symptoms of DEB are less extreme than symptoms of EDs, they still need to be taken seriously. DEB can often be harder to recognize, making it more difficult to know for certain if you should be concerned, making it easier to doubt yourself as a parent.

Dieting is one of the most common forms of disordered eating, and it's much more prevalent among this age group than you might assume. Keep in mind that from an ED lens, *any* kind of dieting is considered disordered eating—even if that diet is considered "healthy." Weight-loss programs and diets don't take into consideration a kid's unique growth and developmental needs and can result in a child feeling hungry, low in mood, and lacking in energy. A child who is dieting may develop poor mental and physical health as well as learning loss and poor concentration.

While there is no one single reason why a child develops DEB, there are two major risk factor categories: the pervasiveness of beauty and diet culture (wanting to look like the models, actors, or influencers they see online or on TV) and preexisting mental health conditions such as depression, anxiety, or OCD, or a family history of mental health issues. If a kid has a higher likelihood due to genetics and is following a lot of beauty influencers online, and then a stressor occurs—it could be puberty, losing a best friend, academic challenges at school—that child may become more vulnerable to DEB. Sometimes the stressor can be a traumatic event such as abuse, neglect, or a car accident. Whatever the source, this stress can trigger the onset of disordered eating patterns, sometimes starting off with a loss of appetite or eating for comfort. If the stress is not addressed or managed, this response can become an unhealthy pattern that can go on for a while before being noticed or addressed.

As Keiran confessed to me, he had a lot of feelings of guilt and shame around his disordered eating. Like many children with DEB, he had issues around control—and in this case, feeling out of control over his weight, body, and food choices. When these out-of-control feelings started to intensify, so did his behaviors, and he started creating rituals and routines around meals and food such as only eating certain foods and not deviating from those foods. Children with DEB will often have an all-or-nothing mindset around "healthy" and low-fat foods.

At the same time Keiran's parents brought him to me, they also took him to his pediatrician, who monitored his weight and blood labs, all of which looked healthy. I spoke with the pediatrician so that we could collaborate on his treatment plan and approach. In our sessions, Keiran and I addressed his issues of control first. To begin with, we worked on rigid patterns that were unrelated to food: I asked him to ride his bike to school a different way and to change the place where he sat and ate his lunch, both good entry points for him to start practicing flexibility in challenging yet achievable ways. We then shifted to mealtimes that his parents could monitor, slowly adding new foods, ones that he historically liked and ate, to breakfast and dinner. While this was gradual, it was consistent, steady and successful.

In our sessions we then discussed related issues such as self-esteem, confidence, and identity. Keiran wanted to be liked and accepted. He wanted to be "really good" at something. He wanted people to think he was funny. He also wanted his family and teachers and peers to think that he was a good person, and not to worry about him. We worked on his relationship with himself, along with his relationship with food, over the course of his sixth-grade year and into the start of the seventh grade. Slowly, Keiran was able to shift out of disordered eating patterns, his self-esteem improved, and he had awareness of his own behavioral patterns. He knew that when he started getting more controlling, that was a signal that something else in his life wasn't going the way he wanted, and he committed to taking the time to figure that out versus going back to old patterns. I told Keiran—when we stress, we regress—and he said he would remind himself of those words when he felt triggered.

Here are some red flags that your child may be engaging in disordered eating:

- **Emotional eating.** It's normal for a child to occasionally lose her appetite when she's feeling low, or to seek comfort in candy when feeling stressed. But as a parent, you'll want to be on alert for when habits shift from a short-term solution in response to an emotional need to more entrenched, repeated behaviors. If your kid comes home on a regular basis and is binging on food or restricting because she's low/stressed, this is a red flag that she's using food as a means to meet emotional needs.
- **Restricting.** Your child starts counting calories, reading food labels, and asking about the fat content of certain foods. At first it may seem like she's educating herself about nutrition, even engaging in healthy habits, but you then discover that she is actually restricting, not just certain foods, but also whole meals, based upon the idea that they might make her gain weight. Hiding food, eating alone, or engaging in secretive behaviors around food consumption can be signs that a child is experiencing shame or guilt related to eating habits. Physical signs such as fatigue, dizziness,

fainting, hair loss, dry skin, or digestive issues can result from inadequate nutrition and restricted food intake.
- **Avoidance.** Your child may start off with restricting a certain food that may seem reasonable based upon a change in appetite or its nutritional value (a candy bar) but then you notice that it leads to avoiding an entire food group (all sweets), then major food groups (all carbohydrates). Irritability, mood swings, anxiety, or depression, particularly around mealtimes or when food is present, may suggest that a child is struggling with disordered eating behaviors. Avoidance of social gatherings or activities that involve food, as well as isolating herself from friends and family, may be a response to disordered eating behaviors and related feelings of shame or embarrassment.

If you notice any of these behaviors in your child, you can approach speaking to her about what you've observed in a nonjudgmental, even tone of voice. You can say, "I notice that you've been avoiding eating certain foods. Tell me about this." Wait to hear what she has to say and show caring and calm concern.

Restricting and other rigid food behaviors can affect a child's physical health, so your first port of call if you're worried about DEB should be your pediatrician. Call in advance to explain your concerns and ask for a physical. Your pediatrician may want to do bloodwork to check for any problems. Once you get the results of the exam, and if indeed your child needs treatment, you may be referred to an ED specialist, typically a master's or doctoral level mental health clinician, who will likely work with a team of clinicians who specialize in ED treatment. This may include a psychologist to provide psychotherapy, a psychiatrist to assess whether prescription medication would be helpful, a registered dietitian to provide guidance and planning on nutrition and meal planning, and a medical or dental specialist to treat health or dental problems that result from some types of EDs.

Although we only very rarely see eating disorders such as anorexia nervosa, binge-eating disorder, and bulimia nervosa in middle childhood, BDD and DEB are both risk factors for EDs, so as a parent, it's so important to be aware of early signs and symptoms, which *often begin in the middle childhood years*. Understanding the gravity of EDs and the importance of intervening as early as possible is critical. According to the NIMH, these complex conditions can impair a person's health and ability to function in everyday life and are "serious and often fatal illnesses that are associated with severe disturbances in people's eating behaviors and related thoughts and emotions."[16]

> ### Picky Eaters
>
> If you're reading this chapter and you have a picky eater at home, you may be wondering if you should be worried. Fortunately, a picky eater is very different from a child with DEB or an ED. A picky eater has identified foods she consistently eats—for instance, she may only eat pasta, white bread, chicken, and a small range of fruits and vegetables. A picky eater typically doesn't want to eat new foods; she prefers what's familiar, and she may not want to even eat familiar foods outside of her home. But a picky eater doesn't binge or deprive herself of those foods—she just eats a normal amount of them and she's consistent in this. The thing about disordered eating is that it's usually inconsistent. A child with DEB may suddenly restrict her diet to include only a small variety of foods, she may compulsively eat a particular kind of food or eat that food very quickly or start to have irregular or inflexible eating patterns. Kids with disordered eating are sometimes uninterested in food, they have a fear of choking, gagging or vomiting when they eat, they may say they aren't hungry or that they are full around mealtimes, and they may not want to eat around other people.

ARFID: The Most Common Eating Disorder in Middle Childhood

Although eating disorders such as anorexia nervosa and bulimia nervosa aren't commonly seen in the middle childhood years, there is one type that we do see, and that's avoidant restrictive food intake disorder (ARFID). A child with ARFID will limit the amount or type of food she eats, but not because she is worried about her weight. She might have sensory issues that cause her to find the smell, texture, or taste of certain foods deeply unpleasant, and so she will refuse to eat them. This is more than just "picky eating." A child with

ARFID may have such an obsession with avoiding certain foods that it can lead to malnutrition. Children with ARFID may become dehydrated, start to lose weight, and fail to grow at the same rate as their peers. This type of ED commonly develops in childhood and can affect adults as well.

Here are some warning signs that your child might be struggling with ARFID:

- Your child consumes only a very narrow range of foods and may refuse even those foods if they appear new or different.
- Your child might need to have the food cut or prepared a certain way in order to eat it.
- Your child is unconcerned about body image issues or weight concerns.
- Your child isn't growing at the same weight as her peers and may have nutritional deficiencies.
- Your child might skip the birthday party or family gathering because she's too stressed about what she's going to eat. She may start to withdraw and not eat with others in general.

If you are concerned that your child is struggling with ARFID, you should know that while this condition is serious, there are helpful and effective interventions. These are best done in collaboration with a professional who is qualified to treat ARFID, such as a licensed eating disorder therapist and/or an occupational therapist. Your pediatrician can help you find someone, and there are support groups online if you're feeling overwhelmed or alone.

Tips for Picky Eaters

Remember that picky eating is sometimes "developmentally normal," especially in very young children. Kids across the globe go through a picky eating phase from about age two to age four. If your child is age six and up and still picky, here are some suggestions to consider:

- Offer her a variety of foods, and give her choices, so she can feel more control over what she eats.

- Serve new foods with established foods that you know she likes. Start with small bites, licks, or even just smells or touches.
- Be persistent: even if your child rejects the new food the first time, try again, and again, and again, as she may eat it the fifth time you serve it. You might need to introduce a new food to your child between fifteen to thirty times before she can say if she truly doesn't like it, so just stick with it!
- Model eating a variety of food for your child and talk about how much you're enjoying the different tastes, textures, and flavors.
- Involve your child in food shopping, meal prep, and cooking: she may be more likely to eat something new if she's made it herself.
- Celebrate any and all gains made in the moment. Even if she eats one bite of a new food, it's worth praising her for the attempt.
- Try to make mealtimes as enjoyable as possible. Despite the frustration of having a child who is a picky eater, you don't want to turn the dinner table into a battleground.
- If nothing seems to be working, and you have been consistent and persistent, talk to your pediatrician about vitamins, supplements, and when to see a feeding specialist or occupational therapist for treatment. Together, rule out other causes, as children can experience feeding challenges due to sensory issues and/or food allergies.

Childhood Obesity

I first met Ella in third grade. Initially, I started seeing her for behavioral problems. Her parents told me she wouldn't listen to them, she was rude and disrespectful to most other adults, and she didn't get along well with her peers at school. After a couple of weeks of working together, it became clear that Ella was being teased by a group of kids for her weight and that this was significantly contributing to her negative behaviors and outbursts, which I came to understand were also symptoms of depression.

At eight, Ella was entering puberty on the earlier side, a development that only exacerbated her insecurity about her body. She confided in me that one of her lowest moments wasn't even when the mean kids called her names at school but when her grandmother described her as "fat" in front of the whole family at a birthday party. Even months later this memory choked her up. Confirming Ella's fears, at her annual visit to see the pediatrician, her parents were told that her BMI was now at the ninetieth percentile, an increase since the year before from the eighty-fifth percentile, and close to obesity.

Ella isn't alone in her struggles. Childhood obesity[17] is an epidemic in this country, with 21 percent or one out of five children in the US between the ages of six and eleven having obesity, according to the CDC. Due to the inequities between race and poverty, obesity is particularly prevalent among Hispanic and Black children, with one in four being affected. Meanwhile, the number of kids who are aged six to eleven and who are overweight has doubled since the 1980s, and the number of adolescents who are overweight has tripled. There's even a new percentile for weight: the 125th percentile for children who fall outside of the existing measure. On the mental health front, research shows that many people who have obesity also struggle with depression, anxiety, EDs, low self-esteem, discrimination, social isolation, and increased risk for substance abuse such as alcohol and drugs, as well as poor body image.[18] And children who are overweight or obese by the age of six tend to stay overweight or obese when they are adults.

Since June 2023, the AMA has classified obesity as a disease, although the National Institutes of Health (NIH) has categorized it as such since 1998, which is to say that for those struggling with obesity, this is not a question of willpower, lack of exercise, or eating too much. This is a chronic illness that can have a real impact on a child's future health. When I use the terminology "are overweight" or "have obesity" it is because this is the language used by the AMA, NIH, WHO, CDC, and the AAP. All of these entities also categorize obesity as a disease because, simply put, it increases the risk of other physical health issues such as sleep apnea, joint pain, high blood pressure, high cholesterol, high triglycerides, type 2 diabetes, heart disease, breathing problems, cancer, a host of metabolic disorders, and ultimately premature death. As a result of the prevalence and seriousness of this public health concern, the AMA issued new guidelines in 2023 around the treatment of childhood obesity, calling for earlier and more aggressive interventions. Although many advocates have pushed back against these recommendations, insisting they will increase weight stigma and eating disorders, as a pediatric psychologist, I can say that these recommendations have sounded an alarm for me around the importance of being proactive in cases where I feel a child may be at risk of health problems down the line due to weight.

As I explained to Ella's parents, obesity is a highly complex issue with a lot of contributing factors. What you eat and how much you exercise is only one part of the picture. Obesity runs in families—this was true of Ella's family—and so genetics play a large part, as does your environment, including the quality of your nutrition, your socioeconomic status, and your experiences during early life. Even higher levels of maternal stress while in utero can play a role. Social and emotional factors, including peer influences and self-esteem, may contribute to food choices, overeating, or being less involved socially or athletically, which may result in a sedentary lifestyle. And even with this complex list of factors, you can have children in the same family, exposed to a similar environment, with one who more easily gains weight while the other does not.

For kids in middle childhood, the hormonal changes of puberty are also a risk factor in obesity as they were for Ella. The hormones leptin and insulin, sex hormones, and growth hormones can influence a child's appetite, metabolism, and body fat distribution. When a child goes through earlier puberty her body may start to store more fat tissue, which can affect her overall body composition and health. During this period, a child's body is preparing for growth spurts that require additional energy and nutrients, leading to increases in height, bone density, and muscle mass. Girls typically experience an increase in body fat in preparation for reproductive health, while boys gain muscle mass and bone density. Changes in eating habits and appetite may also occur, as these hormonal shifts affect hunger, cravings, and food preferences.[19] The longer the pubertal window and the earlier puberty begins, the greater the risk of obesity.

Thankfully, Ella's parents recognized that they were dealing with a potentially serious health issue for their daughter, and they wanted to do whatever they could to help. I suggested we partner with a team at the children's hospital's weight management program, who are experts in guiding families on these issues—and so that's what we did. Ella's parents were surprised to hear that, along with the hospital team, I didn't advocate for putting Ella on a restrictive diet. Her mother understandably reacted to the news that Ella was being fat-shamed in elementary school by wanting to replace all sugar and junk foods in the house with fruits and vegetables so that Ella would lose weight. I explained to her that being reactive was not advised, that it could lead to Ella engaging in disordered eating, and instead we worked together as a team to create a more holistic approach to her daughter's treatment plan.

Today's guidance is that most foods are on the table for kids and that parents need to put the emphasis on *a balanced approach that encourages moderation and establishing healthy eating habits* rather than getting fixated on restricting foods and thinness. In line with the advice of the hospital team, I cautioned it was going to be very important *not* to refer to "good foods," and "bad foods" in front of Ella. Instead, the parents should talk about how there's "some foods we're going to have a lot of the time in our house" (fruits, veggies, whole grains, proteins) and "there's some foods we're going to have a little of in our house (highly processed food such as candy and chips). I encouraged them to bring this up in matter-of-fact conversations over dinner about how certain foods affect our energy, brains, and overall sense of well-being.

Together with the hospital team, I also advised the parents to get Ella involved in a range of after-school activities. She joined a beginner tennis program, which met twice a week. The whole family started going on bike rides on weekends. Two days a week they went to the local rec center pool for open swim time and lessons. Ella also joined a Girl Scout troop where she found a very accepting group of girls, which helped to boost her self-esteem and confidence. Ella's mom spoke to the troop leaders and told them what had been going on at school. These experienced and compassionate leaders made inclusivity a part of the lessons, which created a space for the girls to talk about their experiences of being left out or misunderstood. I also worked with this family on strategies for helping Ella stand up to the kids at school while collaborating with her teachers to help address this kind of cruelty and discrimination.

As I explained to Ella's parents, the most important thing they could do to support their daughter in this situation was to send her a consistent message about accepting and loving herself, without stigmatizing or shaming her. I counseled them to remind Ella of all her innate qualities: that she's an amazing friend, a loving daughter, and hardworking student. It was so important that Ella understood that her weight didn't define her and, at the same time, that eating in a balanced way and spending time moving her body were important: "You can love who you are while also doing things like eating well, exercising, seeing friends, taking part in a variety of activities, all of which keep us healthy."

Ella lost a significant amount of weight over the course of fifteen months. Throughout her treatment we put the emphasis on feeling good and physically doing more. She learned to stop hating her body, began to accept that everyone's bodies are different shapes and sizes, and that the most important thing was that she felt better and was involved in activities that boosted her happiness and her health.

Although weight gain during puberty is normal and necessary for healthy development, if you're at all worried about where your child falls on the growth chart, my recommendation would be not to wait until your child's next well visit. Make an appointment now, then call ahead and give your pediatrician the heads-up that you would like to discuss this topic during the visit. If you feel that your doctor shames or stigmatizes your child for her weight during the visit, you should feel empowered to change physicians. If you decide that you would like specialist help, do your research and ask around for a reputable treatment provider. Many more practitioners are now using telehealth, which may make a specialist who isn't in your area viable for you.

The good news is that for children in the six to twelve age range, focusing on nutrition, exercise, and behavior modification, as well as modifying the kinds of food that are kept in the home, can be successful, as they were for Ella. Guiding a child to understand hunger and fullness cues and understanding the emotions that may trigger her eating habits can also have a big impact. Studies have shown that a family approach where the whole family eats the same food is best, as it sends the message that you aren't eating certain things because you are on a diet, but rather because it is what's healthy for the whole family.

Processed and Ultra-Processed Food

A lot has been written about the detrimental effects of processed and ultra-processed food (UPFs). UPFs include packaged snacks, some chips, processed meats, soda, candy, chocolate, cereal, fast food, and frozen meals that are usually high in sugar, sodium, preservatives, trans fats, and artificial colors. As such they've been linked to a variety of diseases including obesity, mental health disorders, cardiovascular disease, type 2 diabetes, and even premature death.[20]

They may even have a connection to the phenomenon of earlier puberty in children. Research indicates that diets high in these types of foods can lead to excessive weight gain and obesity, which are risk factors for earlier puberty. Excess body fat affects hormone levels, including insulin and estrogen. Metabolic processes also appear to be influenced by the high levels of additives found in UPFs. While there is growing evidence of these associations, we don't fully understand them, and further research is needed.

In addition to the earlier puberty and physical health risks, there seem to be links between UPFs and mental health issues.[21] Adults reporting higher intakes of UPFs were *significantly more* likely to report mild depression and greater levels of anxiety. In children, the connection between ultra-processed food and mental health is particularly important due to the critical role of nutrition in early brain development and emotional well-being. While research specifically focused on children is still limited, there appear to be several ways that UPFs may contribute to less optimal brain functioning and mental health challenges in children including nutritional deficiencies, unstable blood sugar, poor gut health, hyperarousal, and inflammation that interfere with focus, concentration, mood, sleep, appetite, and overall brain health. Unfortunately, because UPFs are widely available, less expensive, flavorful, and fast—and because about 6 percent of American families live in food deserts[22] where fresh and whole foods aren't widely available, the NIH calculates that American kids and teenagers have diets that include close to 70 percent UPFs.[23]

Whole foods consist of fruits, vegetables, whole grains, legumes, fish, shellfish, eggs, and unprocessed meats, as long as they are kept in their natural form and nothing (or very little) is changed or added so that the nutrients in the food remain intact.

Minimally processed foods are foods that have been changed from their original form in some way. Most foods we eat have undergone some degree of processing, whether it's washing, chopping, drying, freezing, or canning, and that's not necessarily a bad thing; in fact it can be a good thing.

Processed foods have been changed from their original form in some way with a few added ingredients.

Ultra-processed foods (UPFs) are any foods that have been through industrial processes changing them from their natural state until they're unrecognizable from how they started. These foods usually have additives, preservatives, sugar, salt, coloring, flavoring, and other artificial ingredients.

Tips for identifying UPFs:

- If this is new to you, don't worry, UFPs are actually pretty easy to spot: they're the ones with long ingredient lists. In the supermarket, you can find them on shelves or in freezers, refrigerated sections, delis, or bakeries.
- Check to see if the list of ingredients contains at least one item of food never or rarely seen in kitchens (such as high-fructose corn syrup, hydrogenated oils, and hydrolyzed proteins), or classes of additives designed to make the food more appealing (such as flavors, colors, emulsifiers, sweeteners, and thickeners).
- If there is an ingredient you can't pronounce or define, or have never heard of, it's likely a UPF.
- Canned or instant soup, hot dogs, chicken nuggets, white bread, French fries, chips, candy, ice cream, cereal, deli meat, sausage, frozen pizza, crackers, and baked goods are common UPFs that are fed to kids.
- While this is not a hard-and-fast rule, a general rule of thumb is that **five** or more ingredients means it's likely a UPF.

A Note on Sugar

Yes, you should try to reduce sugar whenever possible. Studies show that the majority of Americans consume three times the recommended level of added sugar in their day-to-day diets, with sweet foods and drinks making up three-quarters of that. The AAP recommends that kids over the age of two have less than twenty-five grams of added sugar each day (around two tablespoons). Meanwhile, a study out of UC San Francisco published in 2016 found that cutting sugar from kids' diets improved their health in just nine days.[24] After just nine days on the sugar-restricted diet, virtually every aspect of the participants' metabolic health improved, without a change in weight. Studies also show that too much sugar can exacerbate depressive symptoms in people.

Tips for All Kids Around Body Image and Food

As a parent, it can be very difficult to strike the right balance when speaking about body image and food in your home, regardless of your child's weight. There is a lot of stigma about food and body image out there in the world already and you don't want to add to it. Open communication is key, as is being clear and consistent about nutrition and movement routines.

Here are some ideas for how to do this:

- **Promote health, not appearance.** When you emphasize the importance of nutritious eating, hydration, and regular physical activity, your focus should be on overall well-being as the goal, rather than appearance. Don't say, "Let's go for a bike ride together, we need to work off the fat we put on over the holidays . . ." Instead say, "Let's go for a bike ride together, we need to get the endorphins flowing: they're our feel-good chemicals!"
- **Avoid talking about dieting and weight.** Whatever you do, try to avoid discussing diets, weight loss, or other appearance-focused topics that may contribute to unhealthy body image in front of your child. The younger you can encourage a healthy and balanced relationship with food, the better children seem to do as they grow older. Put the focus on lifestyle choices that allow you and your child to do the things that you enjoy. Instead of saying, "I can't have the muffin for breakfast, gotta get rid of my muffin top!" say, "When I have a smoothie, I feel energized until lunch!"

- **Do not put your child on a restrictive diet and don't expose her to weight-loss apps or programs marketed to young people.** As much as you can, avoid messages that encourage restrictive eating. Remember *extreme behaviors, compulsive eating, rigid rules, inflexible eating patterns* are considered restrictive eating and can be detrimental to a young child's health. Be highly cautious of weight-loss apps or online programs marketed for children.
- **Keep less ultra-processed and sugary foods in your house and put the emphasis on moderation.** If your kid is overweight or has obesity, then limiting but not restricting the amount of ultra-processed food and high-sugar food you keep at home is a particularly helpful tip for you. As discussed, these types of foods have been shown to adversely affect children's health. Encourage the idea that many foods can be enjoyed in moderation, which helps prevent the development of an "all-or-nothing" mindset.
- **Talk to your child about the importance of eating meals.** If your child is snacking a lot between meals and then isn't eating as much dinner you can say, "I notice that instead of eating a full meal you're snacking before dinner, which means you are eating less vegetables and protein." It may be that you need to serve your child dinner at an earlier hour to avoid her snacking before the meal.
- **Don't force your child to finish her whole plate.** I grew up this way, and you may have as well. But research shows that you shouldn't force your child to finish her whole plate. Instead, guide her to listen to her body and recognize when she's full, which can help prevent future overeating. This practice is a part of what is referred to as "intuitive eating,"[25] an approach that's about trusting your body to make food choices that feel good for you, without judging yourself or being influenced by diet culture. If your child struggles to finish the food on her plate, try giving her a smaller portion. If she wants more food, she can get more.
- **Avoid food judgment, use neutral language around food, and encourage a balanced approach.** By avoiding negative language around food, you can help your child build positive associations with eating. This can contribute to a healthier relationship with food, reducing the likelihood of guilt or shame associated with certain food choices. Instead of categorizing foods as "good" or "bad," focus on presenting a wide variety of foods as part of a balanced diet. Instead of saying something like "Let's make

healthy choices, eat your vegetables, no more sugar today!" try to use neutral language like "You know, there's a whole bunch of different flavors and textures of food waiting to be explored. Some are crunchy, some are soft, some are sweet, others are salty. Some foods we have as meals, some we have as snacks. Some foods we try to have a lot of and some we have less often." In this way you can emphasize the nutritional value of fruits and vegetables without implying that other foods are inferior.

- **Food as fuel.** Explain that food and water are "fuel for the engine of the body." If your kid understands how computers work, you could try saying, "A computer's CPU needs electricity to function, just like our bodies need food and water to operate efficiently." If your child loves fantasy, explain that food and water are "the wizard making the magic happen." Analogies can help simplify complex concepts and make them more accessible for kids. Once your child understands the concept of food and water as fuel, this will help her make decisions not just based on her body but on her *brain's* functioning. And what's good for the brain is good for the body. Proper nutrition, stimulation, and a supportive environment are crucial for optimal brain development, especially during childhood.
- **Explain "food mood" to your child.** Balanced meals provide us with increased energy, improved concentration, less irritability, better sleep, and a regulated mood. Talk to your kid so she's aware of this, but keep your language neutral and nonjudgmental. Instead of saying, "Don't eat junk food all night at the sleepover! It's so bad for you! You'll be a disaster tomorrow!" say, "I know you're going on a sleepover, just be mindful of how much candy you eat late at night, it might keep you awake, and it will affect your mood tomorrow if you don't sleep well."
- **Teach your child about how our emotions can sometimes send us messages via our body about whether it's time to eat or not.** For example, when we're in a stress state, there is a physiological, not just psychological, response. The fight, flight, or freeze response is activated, the muscles in the abdomen contract, and blood flow increases in the extremities to help us fight back or run away from danger. In order to perform these protective responses, the GI system organs, including the stomach, tense up, allowing the body to do what it needs to do to protect us. Hence, we don't tend to feel hungry when we're in a stress response. It's evolutionary! So if your kid loses their appetite, consider checking to see if they're

feeling stressed. In the same way, if we feel lonely, we might feel a pit in our stomach, then eat a tub of ice cream to fill that void. The solution to this kind of response is to identify the action that best meets the need. For example, you can say to your child: "When I feel lonely, I reach for a hug from loved ones instead of reaching for food when I know I'm already full."

While you are doing your best to establish a healthy relationship for your child between food and body image, remember that what we model is highly influential to children in this stage. So, whether that is talking about pounds on a scale, calories in food, or rushing through meals, they are watching and learning. This topic can be an emotional one for parents who struggled with their weight as a child or do now.

Food Responsiveness

What It Means and How to Identity It

Food responsiveness is a term in psychology that describes the strong urge to eat when you see or smell food. A 2024 report in *The Lancet Child & Adolescent Health* found that kids ages four or five with "higher food responsiveness" went on to have a greater likelihood of self-reported EDs in their late tween and early teen years.[26] When kids with this trait smell or see food—even if it's in a video or photo—they may eat a greater amount in response than other children. They might find it harder to resist snacking and control portion sizes. This can lead to overeating and weight gain, especially if they live in a home with readily accessible prepackaged foods. Both genetics and environment are thought to play a role in food responsiveness.[27]

Looking Ahead

Research shows that eating disorder symptoms are most likely to start between the ages of twelve to twenty-five. While girls in this age range are significantly more likely to struggle with an eating disorder, adolescent boys are also vulnerable. Body image issues peak in adolescence. It's likely that in the next few years your daughter may tell you she wishes she could be skinnier or prettier, or your son may tell you he wants to be taller or more muscular. Rather than being caught off guard, you will be prepared for how to respond: challenging current beauty standards, explaining that images in the media are often unrealistic and unattainable for most people, and encouraging your child to question these standards and to redefine beauty on her own terms. Beauty culture will impact each teen to varying degrees. With intentional guidance, open communication, and fostering a shared understanding about relationship with food and body image in these early years, you're equipping yourself with the means to either prevent or address any red flags that may arise with your child in the future.

In a Nutshell

At this young age, your child is still looking to you for guidance about how to think about her body and how she eats. When you are mindful and intentional about how *you* think and talk about body image and food around her, you have a golden opportunity to help her develop healthy habits and a positive relationship with her body and food. You can help steer her in the right direction if you keep the following in mind:

- Be aware that body image issues and disordered eating can happen for children in this age group, both boys and girls.
- Understand that puberty can be a risk period for body image, disordered eating, and obesity.
- Foster self-esteem in your child as a safeguard against body image issues.
- Avoid commenting on children's size or shape, even if you're complimenting her positively.
- Be a good role model for your child around food and body image. Don't talk about dieting or how you want to "shed the pounds."
- Be on alert for warning signs that your child may be struggling with body image issues or disordered eating.

- If you're worried that your child may be having issues, raise it with her in a gentle, nonjudgmental way.
- Understand body shaming. Work with your child if she is being bullied in this way.
- Don't ban sugar and highly processed foods from your home, but limit them.
- Don't refer to "good" foods and "bad" foods—instead talk about eating in a balanced way.
- Seek out opportunities to add more fresh whole foods or increase enjoyable movement.
- Understand that obesity is a disease. It's not necessarily anyone's fault, but it *is* a significant health issue.
- Don't put your child on a diet.
- Don't force your child to finish what's on her plate.
- Teach your child about mindful eating: encourage her to listen to fullness and hunger cues.
- Talk to her about food as fuel.
- Make the connection for her between food and feelings.
- Eat dinner and cook with your child as often as you can.
- Seek support for yourself and your child if necessary.

CHAPTER 8

Preteens and Success

Shaping Healthier Digital Habits

> We have age restrictions on smoking, gambling and alcohol, and we have no age restriction on social media and cell phones which is the equivalent of opening up the liquor cabinet and saying to our teenagers . . . by the way if this adolescence thing . . . if it gets you down . . .
>
> —Simon Sinek

These days, if you're a parent, screens are going to be part of your family's story. In my practice, it doesn't matter who I'm working with, or the reason they originally came to me, screens *always* come up in our sessions. Parents are frustrated: they don't want their kids to spend so much time on screens, but they feel like the bad guy, always policing their children. And children are just as upset. They say they need their computer for schoolwork or educational apps, that their friends are starting group chats and playing video games together after school and that if they didn't have access they'd feel left out. Screen use pits parents and kids against each other and can feel like a digital tug-of-war that doesn't end.

One parent in my practice struggling with this issue, Jon, had recently gone through a divorce and was in the process of getting remarried. His two kids, aged nine and eleven, were angry at him, and he felt he was no longer able to connect with them in any meaningful way.

"They don't want to spend time with me," he said, clearly upset. "They just want to be on YouTube or video games all the time. I'm trying to make things better, but I'm running up against a brick wall. I just don't know what to do anymore."

I decided to tell him about another family I knew who had just had one of the best trips they could recall to Bryce Canyon National Park. "They made the decision to go screen-free for a week," I explained. "No wi-fi, no phones or iPads, just being together in nature, camping." During the trip, their twelve-year-old, who was usually a moody kid—who typically spent hours a day playing video games—experienced a complete transformation. "He was back to smiling, laughing, and goofing around with his parents," I described to Jon. "It was like he became a fully functioning kid after just twenty-four hours off screens."

Jon had an immediate and positive reaction to the idea of a no-screens break: "That's what I'm going to do with my kids," he told me. "I'm going to take them away for spring break, so we can be together, and we're going to leave the screens behind. I just want our relationship to improve; that's all I want in the world." Even thinking about this trip made his eyes well up with tears. Even though he wasn't sure if he could really get his nine- and eleven-year-old to do this without hating him, he was determined to give it a try. He felt like his relationship with them depended on it.

About a week after they got back, we had a session, and I asked him how it went.

"We did it!" he said, obviously elated. "We did bring the devices, but they were shut down and put away all day. I gave the kids thirty minutes a night to look at their iPads or phones and that was it. I followed the same rules: no more than thirty minutes for me either. We actually played cards and board games together; we read books, stared at the stars, and hiked because there was nothing drawing them inside; we swung in hammocks and looked up at the clouds and the shapes they made; we actually made eye contact and talked at meals. We did it!"

He had assumed that his kids would be furious with him for limiting their screen use; and that they would go back to their mom and tell her that they had a terrible time. But after the initial whining was over, he could tell that they enjoyed just being kids again. The rules were simple and clear, and they followed them—as did he. The dedicated time enabled his kids to open up in ways they hadn't before. On a hike, his daughter opened up about some of the feelings she had about his upcoming wedding, and her worries that it would mean her dad would no longer want to spend as much time with her—and he was able to reassure her that this wasn't going to be the case. "I was shocked that going screen-free made such a big difference," he told me, "but it worked. We connected again."

In the past twenty years, we have gone through a major transformation in our habits as human beings. We've left behind a world that was largely analog to one where everything takes place online. Today, you can barely even look at a menu in a restaurant or pay to park your car or get on a bus without a smartphone. And just as adults have had to change and adapt to this new way of living, the definition of childhood has shifted too. In the past, being a kid meant spending time outside, riding bikes, playing in parks, and running around with other kids or siblings. These times were marked by protected innocence, the freedom to explore and the ability to be creative without anyone tracking you. This seemingly simple childhood allowed an entire generation from the 1990s and earlier to play a significant role in shaping limitless innovation that stimulated the tech boom that would follow. Now time outside running through sprinklers, picking dandelions, and making up street games has been replaced by group chats, memes, filters, and gaming online, inside, and alone.

Screen use today starts when children are toddlers with educational shows and cartoons on iPads, then it progresses to playing simple digital games in preschool, then watching videos online in kindergarten. Even art has gone from paint brushes to a stylus pen on a tablet that needs to be charged before use. By third grade, the great divide begins. Some kids still have limited screen use, but many now have console games, unrestricted YouTube, and social games like Roblox. In the US, on average, **children have their first smartphone by age ten** and nearly three-quarters own a smartphone by age twelve. And before long, kids are spending the majority of their free time on their Instagram, TikTok, and Snapchat accounts. From 2019 to 2021, daily screen use among kids ages eight to twelve grew from four hours and forty-four minutes a day to five hours and thirty-three minutes.[1] According to a study published in the journal *Nature*, children now spend half as much time outdoors as their parents did.

When smartphones and social media first arrived in our lives, we didn't always have all the information we needed to ascertain how harmful these new platforms might be for kids. I remember back in 2010 doing a segment for a local news station when Instagram was still new, and people were getting concerned about its effects on children because of its beauty filters. At that time, I recall saying that although we didn't have the data yet, it was clear to me where this was headed: filters were not going to be good for kids' self-esteem, especially during the adolescent years. Today, we *do* have the data and it is unequivocal: screen use, and social media in particular, is impairing to kids. In 2023, US Surgeon General Vivek Murthy, the nation's doctor, said that children who are thirteen—the age platforms like YouTube, Snapchat, and TikTok allow kids to join—are too young for social media and that they should wait until age sixteen. In 2024, Dr. Murthy advised placing warning labels, similar to the ones on tobacco products, on social media apps.

"Teens who use social media for more than three hours a day face double the risk of depression and anxiety symptoms, which is particularly concerning given that the average amount of time that kids use social media is three and a half hours a day," Dr. Murthy declared, calling youth mental health "the defining public health issue of our time."

Although Dr. Murthy specifically called out the effects of social media on teens, this is still something that you need to be aware of as a parent of a preteen. A 2023 survey found that **40 percent of eight to twelve-year-olds are already on social media**, regardless of age restrictions on the platforms.[2] Even if you haven't signed up your kid for a social media account yet, your child is likely on YouTube, where kids can watch content fed to them by an algorithm, and where they can comment, share, and create their own content, just like on TikTok. And according to a survey of two thousand US children ages two to twelve, 85 percent said they used YouTube to access videos, making the platform more popular than Nickelodeon, Cartoon Network, Disney channel, Netflix, and all the rest.[3]

We cannot ignore the fact that, as psychologist Jean Twenge has demonstrated through her careful analysis of the data, use of digital media is harmful to children. Around 2012, Twenge wrote, she had noticed that teen sadness and anxiety began to steadily rise in the US and other rich developed countries. She looked for explanations and realized that 2012 was precisely when the share of Americans who owned a smartphone surpassed 50 percent and mobile social media use spiked. Now we know that the result is that kids who use social media spend less in-person time with peers, feel lonelier, and become more vulnerable to unfavorably comparing themselves with others.

Further studies show that widespread social media use coincides with the rise in rates of youth depression and suicide. This isn't just an American problem. It shows up in other countries around the world. In 2019, the WHO published strict guidelines about children's screen time, announcing a law permitting schools to restrict smartphone usage, after results were published implicating intensive digital media use in reducing working memory capacity; in psychological problems, from depression to anxiety and sleep disorders; and in influencing the level of text comprehension while reading on screens.

Right when kids are trying to figure out what they are good at and emerging into a sense of their own identity, they are accessing five and a half hours a day of social media and screen time that we know is highly addictive, continuously rewarding like a slot machine, and detrimental to sleep, physical activity, and attention. It is no surprise that when they enter adolescence and high school, they're ill-equipped to manage stress in real life, with real feelings face to face. When they feel stressed, they regress into what they have been using to cope with boredom, hurt feelings, or entertainment—screens of highly filtered, violent, unrealistic portrayals of modified life—and this gets hard wired into their brain as a coping mechanism.

As a child enters early adolescence, this is a particularly important time for brain development, when brain areas involved in emotional and social aspects (the limbic system) are undergoing intensive changes. Social media in particular may have a profound effect on the adolescent brain: the intensity of social media use has been linked to a different mode of processing emotions in adolescents, as shown in the gray matter volume of the amygdala, the seat of our emotions in the brain. This suggests an important link between social experiences in online social networks and brain development. The interplay between the amygdala and the prefrontal cortex, along with other limbic structures, is crucial for emotional regulation and social skills. Dysfunction in these brain regions can contribute to various emotional and social disorders, such as anxiety disorders, mood disorders, and antisocial behavior. What's more, the fact that children's minds are still developing might make them particularly vulnerable to the kinds of fake or shocking news that often show up online, as well leading them to have unrealistic expectations of themselves, without being able to effectively regulate their emotions.

Studies show us that touch screens actually change our brain, reorganizing the somatosensory cortex, the region of the brain that processes touch. And as the brain has a limited amount of cortical space, engaging in screen-based activities may occupy this space at the expense of activities that require motor coordination and movement. When kids are on screens, they're not spending time developing motor skills through play, sports, or other physical activities and so this sedentary behavior may lead to decreased muscle strength, coordination, and overall physical fitness. Researchers have also discovered that social media use is contributing to an increase in functional movement disorders such as tics.

Perhaps most tragically, screens are costing our kids their childhoods: time that they could be spending acquiring basic skills like practicing taking turns, sharing, compromising, and listening to each other's ideas; experiences they can only obtain while playing in real life with other kids. Combine concerns about screen use and its impact on developing brains and bodies with other well-founded worries about cyberbullying, sexual harassment, and distraction issues that happen online, and you understand why so many parents, educators, and political leaders are up in arms. California, Utah, and other states have passed laws to protect kids from social media. New York City has already declared social media a public-safety hazard for youth mental health.[4] But parents cannot wait for others to act or for such laws to survive legal challenges and take effect.[5]

Here's how I think about this issue: not so long ago, people in this country and around the world smoked cigarettes. Although there were earlier studies indicating that smoking led to lung cancer and other fatal health issues, the US surgeon general didn't release the first report on the health effects of smoking until 1964—and very slowly, over time, the federal government began printing warnings on cigarettes, restricting advertising, and raising the legal age for purchase. In the same way, car seats used to be optional for little kids, even though evidence supporting the protective effect of child restraint devices was available in the early 1970s—and still, laws requiring their use were not adopted by all fifty states until 1986. The same thing is happening here with screens. We know they're harming our children, and now it's time to act.

If you're reading this and your child is six years old, it's likely he's not on social media yet. You may already be dealing with too much screen time and video games, but you still have a chance to prevent low self-esteem, depression, anxiety, eating disorders, and body image issues that may be ahead. We have the data; we must respond the way we do to other things that are harmful, giving our children the time they need offline to be able to grow up safely.

And so, although I know screens are the cause of so much conflict and despair in families, I'm here to give you some hope. If your kid does not yet own a phone, or if they're not on social media, or if they are new to it, you can set the tone starting today. You can delay their access to these devices and apps. And when you decide to allow them, you can set limits and restrictions on how much they can use. Parental controls on devices and apps are now robust: every major device, app, or game on the market these days comes with parental restrictions where you can set time limits and control content and spending. When you use these settings, this has the benefit of making the app or game the bad guy. "I'm sorry kid, that's how much screen time you have today, I can't extend it any further. One of my values is to keep you safe and healthy, that's why I'm setting these restrictions for you."

And just like Jon, the dad at the beginning of this chapter, you can, and you should, designate screen-free time together, taking screens away at certain hours of the day and setting screen-free zones and times for everyone—adults included. Your kids may not thank you for it now, but they will benefit from it later—and so will you.

Here are my suggestions for screen-free zones and times:

- **The dinner table:** Mealtimes are for connecting, sharing, and enjoying food. Screens at a dinner table are attention and relationship disruptors.
- **Bedrooms:** Keep screens out of bedrooms. Bedrooms should be places for sleeping and relaxing, not scrolling.
- **Sleepovers and playdates:** If there are screens when your child is socializing, limit their use and physically take them away when time is up.
- **Vacations:** Consider taking screen-restricted vacations where you commit to following the same rules as your kids.
- **Family game nights:** Set nights of the week where you play offline games like charades, Twister, or cards, or do puzzles together.
- **Time with family and friends:** Your children need time to connect with family and friends in real life. Devices away = play.

In this chapter, I'm going to look at how we, as parents, can be proactive about delaying, limiting, and monitoring our children's screen use. Many books have already been written about how harmful screens are, but my goal is to give you practical, actionable advice so that you can prevent screens from becoming a battleground for your family during this crucial period of your child's development.

> **PARADIGM SHIFT**
>
> **Paradigm:** Screens are just part of our lives now. I know they're bad for children, but all their friends are on screens, they have to do their schoolwork and homework on screens, they say they will be left out if they don't have certain apps; there's not really much I can do about it.
>
> **Shift:** Screens have detrimental outcomes for children, and you *can* do something about it. Companies are responding to parents' advocacy on this issue and are putting in place guardrails that you can use to limit, restrict, and control your child's screen use. Don't expect your child to be able to limit his own use—it's far too addictive for kids to control on their own. It's your job to teach and model moderation. With an investment of your time and energy, you can set your child up for a successful and better-balanced relationship with technology. This is hard—but it's not impossible.

Sound Familiar?

- Your child is at the age where he's asking for more and more screen time, but you don't feel ready for him to be exposed to everything that comes along with that.
- Your child's peers are already getting phones and gaming consoles, and you feel the pressure from your child to do the same.
- You want to restrict how much screen time your kid has but feel overwhelmed by how homework, downtime, and even socializing is now digital, whether on smartphones, tablets, or gaming consoles.

- Your child's peers are allowed a lot of screen time, and you feel pressure to allow more screen time than you're comfortable with.
- You're not sure if all screen time is created equal. You wonder if your kid playing an educational game on a laptop is better than watching an educational show on a tablet.
- You feel like you can't possibly monitor all the content your kid can be exposed to. They may be watching a show on YouTube one minute and then getting alerts on a group chat the next.
- You are exhausted by setting limits on screen time that your kid constantly pushes up against, negotiates, or just ignores.
- You know you're inconsistent with the amount of screen time your kid has; it depends on the day, your workload, or how much attention you are paying to the time, but you don't feel like you can keep track of it all.
- Your kid knows how to get around on the internet better than you do, and you feel behind in keeping up with technology.
- At times you feel guilty about how much screen time your kid is getting, but you haven't figured out how to get things done, find time for yourself, and limit their screen time.
- Even though you don't want to overuse the screen as a babysitter and you try to get your kid to go outside and play or do something else, his resistance wears you down.
- You notice your kid is irritable and grumpy when he gets off a screen.

Screens and Sleep

Sleep deprivation, disrupted sleep, and dealing with drama at bedtime may be one of the most powerful unintended consequences of the digital age on kids. Screen use is not only affecting the quantity of hours that kids sleep, but the quality too. This has an impact on how they start their school days and their concentration and focus during class—and their moods when they get home exhausted and take it out on their often equally exhausted parents.

Here's the reason screens at nighttime are so stimulating: the light emanating from the screen sends your brain and body the message that it's still daytime. This has the effect of suppressing melatonin—a hormone released in the body when it's dark—which has the effect of interrupting your body's circadian rhythms, leading to disrupted sleep.

Kids in middle childhood need between nine to twelve hours of sleep every night. Here are my tips for helping your child get a better night's sleep:

- **If your child has a phone, turn off notifications on the device so they're not getting pinged day and night.** A 2023 report from Common Sense Media found that kids and teens are being inundated with phone prompts day and night, with half of eleven- to seventeen-year-olds getting at least 237 notifications a day.[6] Some get nearly five thousand in twenty-four hours.
- **Keep phones and devices out of bedrooms.** My message for kids is: don't sleep with a screen. You wouldn't have someone detoxing sitting in a room with the drug that they are addicted to, and we shouldn't do this to our kids with devices either. Devices should not be charging in your child's bedroom; they should be someplace they can't get access to late at night or early in the morning. And when they tell you they need it in their room as an alarm clock, you can invest a few dollars in an actual, physical alarm clock.
- **Practice digital sundown.** It's a good idea to set time limits on devices so that screens shut down an hour before bedtime, giving kids time to wind down.
- **Change the settings to make screens less bright at night.** Use the Night Shift setting on an iPhone or use the grayscale display on either phone, which minimizes the bright colors that attract and stimulate our brains and keep us on our phones longer. Some people purchase blue light glasses, but we don't have any reliable data to back up the claims that they help prevent eyestrain and sleep problems.

Dopamine 101

It's so important to understand the links between dopamine and screen use, as it helps explain why kids are so magnetically drawn to screens, and why it's so hard for them to get off those screens when you tell them they've had enough. Dopamine is a neurotransmitter in the brain that helps us to feel desire—it's part of the brain's reward system.[7] This explains why we want to do certain things that make us feel good, whether it's playing a video game or eating an ice-cream sundae—activities like these will trigger multiple dopamine rushes in the brain. Dopamine can also affect our ability to learn and pay attention, regulate mood, increase heart rate, and maintain sleep patterns, among other things. Once we get those hits of dopamine, the rush continues; even after your kid gets off the screen or finishes the sundae, the dopamine doesn't immediately fade.

Dopamine is intimately linked to screen use. When your child posts a picture on social media and gets lots of likes and comments, this can give him a dopamine boost. When he keeps scrolling on Instagram, waiting for the next amusing cat video, or funny meme, or outrageous stunt, it's because he wants another reward for his brain's pleasure center. When he's playing video games and he makes it to the end of the round, or levels up, he gets the same kind of hit. This explains why games and social media are so addictive and effective at keeping us coming back for more. Of course a child is going to want more of the rewarding dopamine feeling—his brain has now been primed to expect it. All of this is fine in small doses; the problems start when your child is spending too much time on these dopamine-stimulating experiences. At this point, his reward system will get "hijacked," going into overdrive, which can lead to impulsive and addictive behaviors. Not surprisingly, dopamine plays a part in toxic habits like compulsive gambling and drug and alcohol addiction.

Social media and video game companies understand the role that dopamine plays in keeping us fixated on screens, and they manipulate their products to maximize the amount of pleasure hits we're going to get. When the former vice president of User Growth at Facebook Chamath Palihapitiya sat down with an audience of Stanford students, he admitted feeling "tremendous guilt," about the role he played in exploiting consumers who became hooked on Facebook and other social media sites. "The short-term, dopamine-driven feedback loops that we have created are destroying how society works," he explained, drawing a direct link between social media use and addiction, and the ways that these products are stimulating the same pleasure centers as recreational drugs or gambling.

One way that you can decide if screen time—or anything else—is good for your child is by watching the way he acts afterward. If he's irritable or combative after watching YouTube or playing Fortnite, it's probably not good for him. If your child is spending a lot of time online, you need to be on alert for behaviors in your child that are impulsive and compulsive. These kinds of kids can also be sensory and thrill seekers: the usual is not enough; they need more (when you take them to the amusement park or county fairground, they need to play more games, win more tickets, pick out more prizes). They get hyper-focused on something and it's hard to break them out of it. If this sounds like your kid, it may be that he's more prone to dopamine dysregulation (not an official diagnosis but rather a set of behaviors that we observe in sensation-seeking kids). If that sounds like I am describing a kid with ADHD, well, both ADHD and gambling have been associated with dysregulation of the brain's dopamine system, which plays a role in reward processing and motivation. Dysfunction in the dopamine system may contribute to difficulties in regulating impulses and seeking out rewarding experiences.

Here's the good news—once a child knows that he can't have access to screens or that the limits are firm and nonnegotiable, the craving for video games, or the mindless scrolling, goes away. He will start doing other things; he will want to do other things. So there is plenty you can do to interrupt the dopamine-cycle and its impact on your child's brain: starting with limiting and restricting use.

Is Screen Time Linked to an Increase in ADHD Diagnoses?

The short answer is yes,[8] and here's some context for my response. First, attention deficit hyperactivity disorder (ADHD), as defined by the *Diagnostic and Statistical Manual of Mental Health Disorders* (DSM-5), is a neurodevelopmental disorder characterized by persistent patterns of inattention and/or hyperactivity-impulsivity that significantly interfere with a person's functioning or development. Kids with ADHD may struggle to maintain attention, follow instructions, organize tasks, and sustain mental effort. They may also display hyperactive and impulsive behaviors such as fidgeting, restlessness, excessive talking, and difficulty waiting their turn. To receive this diagnosis, symptoms must be present before the age of twelve, persist for at least six months, and cause impairment in multiple settings, such as school, work, or home.

This question about the association between screen time and ADHD has been controversial and studies have been inconsistent in their findings. However, in 2023, researchers published the results of a meta-analysis of prior research on the association between screen time and childhood ADHD. Based on the results, the study found a positive correlation between screen time and the *risk* of ADHD. This analysis suggests that excessive screen exposure may significantly contribute to the *development* of ADHD in children. These authors recommended reducing screen time in children to prevent the occurrence of ADHD.

The Cleveland Clinic interpreted results from a separate 2018 study and found that the students who reported using digital media many times a day were more likely than their peers to show these symptoms of inattention, such as difficulty organizing and completing tasks, and hyperactivity-impulsivity, and having trouble sitting still. They went on to say that frequent digital media use can bring out latent symptoms or create behaviors that look like ADHD but do not necessarily *cause* ADHD.

As a practitioner who grew up with a sibling who has ADHD, over the last two decades, I have read about and looked at many different factors that have been thought to contribute to ADHD or ADHD-like symptoms, everything from environmental factors, including exposure to toxins such as lead or prenatal exposure to alcohol or tobacco, to social-emotional factors such as maternal stress during pregnancy, low birth weight, and early childhood trauma. I have followed the data on abnormalities in brain development, diet, and nutrition such as studies that have explored the potential impact of food additives, dyes, sugar, and the benefits of omega-3 fatty acids on ADHD symptoms. The findings have been mixed. But here is what we have done with these suspected risk factors—we have addressed them! Psychologists have spoken about these risk factors with their patients, including suggesting parents provide children with low-sugar, nutritious foods. Given the data on the effects of screens on ADHD-like symptoms, we need to respond the same way with screen time, reducing, monitoring, and delaying screen use if we are at all concerned about this issue.

The Wait Until 8th Pledge

I know that by the time you are reading this, some of your kids will already know how to get around a phone better than you. He may have already logged in hours of FaceTime, YouTube, and online games. But getting him his own smartphone changes things—a lot. If having a phone meant just making audio and video calls and sending the occasional text, this wouldn't be life-changing for your child. But for most families, getting your kid a phone means access to an online world that connects him to strangers and exposes him to, well, just about anything imaginable.

I have been a firm believer in the Wait Until 8th pledge (the final year of middle school) for years now. The problem is there's seemingly only small pockets of parents in certain communities willing to wait. Today, the average age for a child to have their first smartphone is ten years old, with nearly one in four children given phones between the age of five and seven.

Wait Until 8th is a movement that started in 2017 when a group of Texas parents banded together, tired of the pressure to give their kids smartphones too young. The movement they founded "empowers parents to rally together to delay giving children a smartphone until at least the end of 8th grade." Further, Dr. Murthy, the US surgeon general, has urged that teens should wait until age sixteen to get on social media. Given the compelling data on the detrimental effects of screens and social media, parents everywhere are being urged to delay, delay, delay.

When parents unify in this, it decreases the pressure felt by both the kids and the parents, and I have found it to be very effective in small circles of friends. If you're still getting pressure from your child because he wants a device, or if you want him to have a device so you can track him and message with him for safety reasons, you can look into getting him a device without internet access, video games, social media, or other apps. This could be a flip phone, a smartwatch, or another kid-friendly device.

If you hold off giving your child a smartphone, your child will be in a minority, but he won't be alone. Right now, it's only three-quarters of kids under the age of thirteen that have smartphones. That leaves a quarter of kids who don't. And parents have the power to change these numbers.

If You Must: A Guide to Giving Your Child a First Smartphone

I think it's best to "Wait Until 8th" or hold off until age thirteen, to give your child a smartphone. But if you choose to give a smartphone earlier, here is a deeper dive into some important considerations and information.

Deciding to give your child a smartphone is one of the most important parenting decisions you will have made so far in your parenting journey. Once you've given your child a phone, you are going to have to deal with all kinds of time-consuming and frustrating problems and conflicts you have avoided until now.

So, before you go ahead, answer these questions:

1. Why are you considering this? Is it pressure from your child, safety, a fear of your child being left out? Once you've figured out your motives, try to imagine the pros and cons of waiting longer. Do the pros outweigh the cons?
2. Has your child already had a simple phone (a dumb phone that only calls a few people with no internet)? Or a smart watch? Could you try that approach first?
3. Do you have the mental energy to place limits on phone use and follow through on them—including taking the phone away if necessary? Do you have the mental energy to monitor your child's screen use? Do you know how to monitor and control their screen time? If the answer is no, you probably need to wait.
4. Does your child seem likely to be able to follow a new set of rules? Does he seem to have effective coping skills? Is he able to limit distractions? Is he responsible and able to track his belongings? If you answered no to any of these, you probably need to wait.
5. Are you ready to manage your own phone use? A new phone owner will be watching you closely to see how you utilize your time. Again, if the answer is no, you probably need to wait.

If you do decide to go ahead and give your child who is under thirteen a phone—or if you're reading this and you have a child who is going to be thirteen soon—here's my advice for doing this responsibly. I cannot emphasize enough how important it is to set the right tone from day one by talking with your child, and restricting, limiting, and monitoring his phone use. Phones and apps are highly addictive, and you cannot expect your child to control his use on his own.

- Before you give your child a phone, you need to set the device up using every parental control available. You can find these in the phone's settings. Set time limits for phone use: make sure that the phone shuts down at least an hour before bedtime and stays shut off all night. You need to ensure your child will have to request your consent to download apps or make in-app purchases. In the app's privacy settings, make sure you always disable the photo, microphone, and location: and add a password so your child can't change the settings. It's a good idea to also disable any notifications for these apps so your child's phone isn't pinging all the time.
- Install parental monitoring on the phone—most devices and apps now have a "family center" that allows you to have a certain level of control on your child's phone. There are also apps you can purchase that have highly sensitive levels of monitoring activity on your child's phone and apps.
- Make sure you know all of your child's passwords and explain to them that you will access his phone using these passwords so you need to be kept up-to-date if there are any changes.
- Consider starting off by enabling your kid to *only* make phone calls, video calls, and use texts. You can build up from there once your child has proven he can be responsible.
- If he proves to you he's responsible, you can build up to browsing, apps, watching videos, playing games, and taking photos. I advise adding one thing at a time. Monitor how it's going. Don't feel pressured to go faster, and if you aren't comfortable with something, then it's not wise to allow it.
- Put in the time and effort to learn about the apps your child wants to add to the phone, always making sure an app or website is age appropriate. I really like Common Sense Media for this kind of information.

When you've done all of these things, it's time to sit your child down and have a meeting about phone use. Even if you only allow your child to text and make phone and video calls, this will still require guidance and rules. This meeting should be the first of many ongoing talks about phone and online behavior.

Here's what you can say:

> I'm giving you this phone as a privilege. A privilege is something that is earned through making good choices and maintaining trust. There are rules around having a phone. I am monitoring what you do with this phone, and I will take it away if you don't follow the rules. Having a phone is a big responsibility, and we need to work together to keep you safe and happy.
>
> As a first step, I have set up the phone so you can only text and make phone or video calls. If you prove to me that you're responsible, we can talk about adding things like a browser and apps.
>
> I know you are going to want to use your phone to text with friends. This can be a lot of fun, but you will need to follow the rules of digital communication when you're texting. Always treat others with kindness and respect. I don't want you to say anything rude, mean-spirited, or threatening in a text.
>
> You should never text anything negative about someone or share a secret about them. It might be tempting to share a secret someone has told you, but we don't do that. Remember: don't say something to someone on your phone that you wouldn't say to them in person, and treat others as you would wish to be treated.
>
> Think before you send. Whatever you send is out in the universe—whether in a cloud, on a screenshot, or in someone's messages. It will live on forever, even if you regret what you sent. Once you've sent it, it's out of your control and it could be shared by other people.
>
> To start, I want you to only text with friends and family. I don't want you to interact with people on your phone that I don't know. You can only have people we know in your contacts until you're older and more experienced.
>
> Do not ever give out your phone number, address, email, or your school in a text or anywhere else online, it's not secure and could be shared with others that you don't know.

Don't overshare. You're going to be excited to have your phone, and it may be tempting to share all your thoughts and feelings on a text. Maybe you're mad at me, or feel like you hate your teacher, or you want to rant about how dumb your coach is. This is not okay to post or text about these feelings. It will also be tempting to share pictures of all sorts of things like new clothes, your friend who is sleeping over, or your sibling having a meltdown. If you want to talk about these things, you should call someone instead of texting it. If you feel a strong urge to share something, you can always take a break, talk to someone in real life, and then see if you want to share it.

I am setting the phone's sleep timer so it shuts down an hour before bedtime. You won't be allowed to have your phone in your bedroom or at mealtimes. There will be other times when you won't have a phone—during dinner, when family is visiting, and when you're supposed to be doing homework.

After you have started this talk, you will want to get your child to sign an agreement. Yes, a signed agreement ensures that everyone understands the rules and agrees to them—kids and adults alike. This avoids conflict down the road when your child turns to you and says "You never told me that!" or "I didn't know I wasn't supposed to do that!"

The New Rules of the Game: Digital Citizenship and the Twenty-First-Century Child

Having children in today's world means that, even if you hold off on giving your child a smartphone and you restrict their time online, they are *still* going to be digitally connected. They will likely have to do schoolwork online, and much of our entertainment is now accessed via the internet. What that means for us as parents is that we need to keep up with what children are doing online, and we have to teach them basic skills and good habits. If you think about it, allowing your kid to interact with the online world is a lot like dropping him in the middle of a foreign city. You can tell him, "Off you go, I'm leaving you now, please find your way home!" Or, you can say, "Hold my hand, I'm going to help you cross the road, show you the way, and teach you how to read a map." If you let your young child have access to this online world *without* offering any guidance, you're essentially telling him to go get lost in a foreign city, walk out into traffic, and talk to strangers.

My rule of thumb is that if you don't feel ready to talk to your child about how to navigate the online world, then you're not ready for him to spend time there.

Starting at age six, you will need to begin to impart some basic rules of digital literacy. You may feel like you're ill-equipped to guide your child; you're not alone. As a first step, you can ask your child's school what they're doing to teach digital literacy and if you can have access to any materials. If they don't have those materials, there are free resources available online: and you could even be a champion for your school to introduce these. Two free curriculums that I have used are Common Sense Media Digital Literacy and Citizenship and Be Internet Awesome by Google.

I started teaching digital citizenship to six-, seven-, and eight-year-olds in 2018. The following is a collective of what I think you need to know to talk to your child about staying safe online.

DIGITAL CITIZENSHIP

What parents need to know: Digital citizenship refers to the responsible and ethical use of digital technology. It encompasses understanding how to use technology effectively, safely, and responsibly. For parents, this means guiding your children from a young age so that they can understand the concepts and consequences of relevant issues such as respecting others online, protecting personal information, plagiarism, privacy, and safety, while playing their part in creating a positive online culture.

What you should tell your children: "Digital citizenship means being responsible at using the internet, apps, games, tablets and computers. It's like having a super map that helps you do lots of cool things online, like finding information for homework, watching videos, talking with friends and playing games. But it's not just about having fun—it's also about being smart, safe, and respectful to others while you're online. Being a good digital citizen means knowing how to talk with others, it means understanding what privacy means, and how to tell if something is true or not. When you have this super map, it will help keep you on the right track, so you don't get lost or wander onto websites, apps, games, or conversations that you don't have permission to be on."

ONLINE PRIVACY

What parents need to know: Online privacy refers to the control and security that your child may—or may not—have while on his digital device. It means protecting sensitive information such as name and contact, social security numbers, and credit card information, and disabling anything in a device or app that allows your child to interact with strangers. Most devices, accounts, and apps your child may want to use have privacy options built into their settings that you, as a parent, need to learn to use. At the same time, your child needs to be aware that the information he's sharing on a site or app might be collected, stored, and used by its owners—and others. He should also understand the importance of not sharing photos of other people without consent, that this can be a legal issue, not just a matter of respect.

What you should tell your children: "The number one rule of privacy is that you should never give out your phone number, address, or school name to anyone online. If you want to give this information to a friend, you should ask me or give it to them in person. This may seem strange to you as your friends and family know your name, number, school, and home address, but the rules change when you're online. Companies are trying to collect information about you when you're online, and I don't want you to share any information unless you ask first. You also need to understand that before you share any picture or video online that has other people in it, you need to make sure you have the other person's permission (also called 'consent'). It's not okay to assume that person will say yes. It's up to you to ask. In the same way, you should never force anyone to share something they don't want to share online. You need to respect that person's privacy just like you would want them to respect yours."

RELIABLE/UNRELIABLE SOURCES

What parents need to know: Reliable sources are those news reports, scientific facts, or descriptions of events that are fact checked, trustworthy, or written by experts who know what they're talking about. Unreliable sources include information that hasn't gone through any kind of fact-checking process, and it's mostly created by people without any training or background in the topic they're talking about—i.e., most of the stuff you can find online.

Due to the proliferation of poor or unreliable sources online, parents and educators *must* teach children how to identify what's a good source, how to identify less reputable sources, and which sources need to be double-checked before you believe them. Research suggests that children often have difficulty recognizing the credibility of online information and understanding the potential for misinformation and manipulation on digital platforms. They may be more susceptible to believing and internalizing content they encounter online, particularly if it aligns with their existing interests. You know how when you are looking for something or someone to validate what you are thinking, and you suddenly find it? We say things like "It's a sign!" Well, so do kids, and the internet and social media are ripe with content that will align with probably just about anything your kid wants. In order to filter out a lot of the inappropriate content a child might find online, you can use a kid-friendly search engine like Google Kids Space. Even a simple Google account can be set up for a child via the family center so that you can monitor and control what your kid sees and does when he's searching online. However, you may want to still introduce your kid to sources that look reputable, but in fact are full of inaccuracies, so you can show your child the difference between a good source and a bad one—and he can learn the difference. Remember when your child was a toddler and you would say silly things like "Do elephants have bananas as noses?" and your toddler would crack up and shout, "Noooo!" This is the middle childhood version. You can play out online scenarios and say, "Now does that really look like that? Or does that sound like that?" and they should still shout back "Nooo!" Teaching children to question sources, verify information, and consider the intentions behind online posts can empower them to think critically and navigate the digital world more effectively.

What you should tell your children: "Not everything you read about and see online is true. Some of it will look like it's real and true, but it still might not be. We're going to work together to figure out ways to make sure the information you're finding online is accurate and real. We can do this by using special search engines and going to news sites that use journalists. Remember, the best people to listen to online are people who are qualified to speak about that topic: a doctor talking about a medical problem, a NASA scientist describing space travel, a well-known singer talking about music. When you see something online that seems outrageous and makes you feel angry, uncomfortable, or you just can't believe it, the first thing you should ask yourself is: Is this true? Don't share anything until you've double-checked that it's true. We have to have multiple credible sources before we can believe it. You need to put your detective glasses on anytime you're online."

ONLINE GROOMING

What parents need to know: "Online grooming" refers to what happens when an adult builds a relationship with a child online with the intention of exploiting him sexually, emotionally, or financially (sometimes referred to as "sextortion"). Grooming typically involves manipulating a child's trust and confidence through friendly conversations, compliments, and the sharing of personal information. The groomer usually intensifies the level of intimacy and control over time, often leading to requests for inappropriate photos or videos, or attempts to meet in person. How to guard against this? You can begin by enabling safeguards such as not approving certain apps, and making sure your kid's accounts are set to private, meaning he won't be able to interact with strangers. You can also set limits on where and when your child can use a device—especially out of their bedroom. In age-appropriate ways you need to explain to your child that not everyone he may encounter online is who they say they are and that you want him to communicate only with people he knows in real life. This needs to be an ongoing talk as he starts to get involved in social video games and his first social media apps.

What you should tell your children: "The reason why we are keeping your accounts private is because that protects you from getting messages from people you don't know. But if someone who you don't know contacts you or makes a comment (even if it's nice) you should not reply to them. You aren't being rude or mean to that person if you do this, and you don't have to worry about not being polite. If in doubt, you can come to me, and I will help you figure out if this person is someone you should communicate with or not. If someone asks for pictures and personal information you should tell me about it immediately and I will help you block them. I may report them if I am concerned but I won't ever be mad at you for telling me."

ARTIFICIAL INTELLIGENCE (AI)

What parents need to know: (*This section is compliments of OpenAI ChatGPT*) AI refers to the simulation of human intelligence in machines that are programmed to perform tasks that typically require human intelligence, such as learning, problem-solving, decision-making, and natural language processing. Most kids today will encounter AI on multiple platforms, including ChatGPT, which is a free chatbot that you can use to have humanlike conversations to answer a question. Schools are beginning to embrace AI, and they're still figuring out how best use it in the context of education. The reality is that AI is here, and now integrated into social media and search engines. We need to make it part of our digital literacy efforts.

What you should tell your children: "'AI' stands for artificial intelligence is like a super smart robot that can learn and solve problems. The bot is not your friend like your real friends. It's a technology that helps machines and computers do things that typically require human intelligence, such as understanding language, solving problems, or creating art. AI can be found in everyday apps like Alexa, in search engines like Bing, or in video games. While AI can make our lives easier and more fun, it's also important to use it responsibly, whether for fun or in school, and to always think critically about the information and ideas it gives you."

DEEPFAKES

What parents need to know: Deepfakes are when artificial intelligence is used to manipulate images, videos, and audio to create realistic looking but totally fabricated content. This may include swapping faces, mimicking voices, and manipulating facial expressions and gestures so that the people in the video say things they didn't say or do things that they didn't really do. When you're looking at a deepfake, you may not immediately realize it's fake, but you may have an "uncanny" feeling, as if something is off. Deepfakes have raised concerns about their potential to spread misinformation, deceive viewers, and manipulate public opinion. They've been used for entertainment like celebrity impersonations, but also for political propaganda, revenge porn, and other nefarious purposes. Sadly, it's not just high-profile figures who are being affected: deepfakes are creeping into schools too, with students using AI to do things like paste the faces of female students onto pornographic images before uploading those images to a website (as happened at a high school in New Jersey).[9] Efforts are underway to put technology in place to immediately detect and flag deepfakes, as well as to raise awareness about their existence and the potential hazards.

What you should tell your children: "Deepfakes are like magic tricks for videos and pictures, where someone's face can be swapped with someone else's, and you may not even know it. People use special computer programs to make these tricky videos, and they can sometimes be used to make someone look like they're saying or doing things they didn't. To spot a deepfake, look for things that look out of place or seem a little bit off. If you're confused, you can always come to me, and we can figure it out together."

CYBERBULLYING

What parents need to know: Cyberbullying is the most common form of bullying today with 57 percent of school-age or six- to twelve-year-old children saying they've been on the receiving end of abusive comments online.[10] This is a serious issue that can have harmful effects on children's mental health and it can happen on all kinds of different platforms including texts, group chats, social media, and gaming platforms. Cyberbullying can take the form of rude messages and embarrassing images or videos. In my experience, it's a form of bullying that kids often keep secret, hoping it will just go away. For many children, it's worse than playground bullying because hundreds of kids will see the embarrassing photo/video and share it or screenshot it. If one child threatens to post something embarrassing about another child unless that child gives them something or does something, that's extortion. When you allow your child to be on any platform, even texting, you need to talk to him about cyberbullying and explain to him that he can always come to you if he's confused or being targeted. Many kids worry they will lose their privileges if they share with you, so make sure you're clear this won't happen. Don't forget that kids can also bully themselves online, posting negative comments about themselves and inviting other kids to weigh in. This is also considered a form of cyberbullying—and is referred to as digital self-harm.

What you should tell your children: "Now that you're online, you're going to be playing or talking with friends and other people you might not know. You need to do this in a way that keeps you and your friends safe. Bullying is when someone says something mean, threatens to do something hurtful, or tries to make someone do something they don't want to do. Cyberbullying is when the same thing happens online. Someone might send you a message that's mean, or post embarrassing pictures or videos of you. If this happens to you or a friend, you can tell me, you won't get in trouble, and we will figure out what to do about it together. I want you to know that we do not say mean things or post mean things online in our family. That's wrong and we don't allow it. If this happens, there will be consequences; you will get your privileges taken away and you may face punishment at school as well."

VIDEO GAMES

This section was written in collaboration with teenage gamers for accuracy and insight.

The first question most parents ask me on the topic of video games is: Are all video games created equal? The answer is no. Video games vary widely in content, gameplay, and intended audience. They can span genres, platforms, and purposes, and they cover a wide range of themes and content, ranging from family-friendly and educational fun to mature-rated (M) titles featuring violence, explicit language, or adult themes.

The good news is that there are excellent educational video games designed to engage kids in learning in a multitude of subjects. Most US schools now use such games that, played in moderation, can be an engaging tool for supporting your child's learning. Research is mounting that games can be useful for making learning fun and more engaging, enhancing attentional skills, and improving recall and problem-solving skills. While more research is needed before we have a full understanding of the efficacy of educational video games, what is certain is that these games are highly appealing to children and get them interested in math games or reading in ways that other teaching methods typically don't.

Parents also want to know if playing violent video games can lead to kids being more aggressive. Ongoing research that looks at the effects of violent video games offers us mixed results, with some studies showing a risk of increased aggressive behavior, a decrease in empathy, and lower levels of prosocial behavior,[11] while others suggest that the relationship between violent video game exposure and aggressive behavior may be influenced by outside factors such as personality traits, family environment, peer influence, and preexisting levels of aggression. Another study found that those who played high-risk games spent significantly more time playing those games, were more interactive with other players, and had poorer sleep outcomes than non-high-risk gamers. Additionally, playing high-risk games had significantly different social impacts compared to less-risky gaming, including spending more money on games, spending less time on homework and with family, or skipping meals due to gaming. My advice is to watch how your child reacts to playing video games in general. How does he act after he's been playing? Does he easily transition? Does he have varied interests? In this way, you'll know whether your child can tolerate these kinds of games or if they seem to lead to an increase of aggressive behavior.

Perhaps the most important thing for all parents to know about video games is that they're highly addictive. Gaming disorder now is recognized by the WHO in the International Classification of Diseases, and it's included in the DSM-5 as an addictive diagnosis. So you do need to be mindful of how much time your child is spending playing these games, who he's playing with, and what the game is actually about. Again, for ages six to twelve, the AAP recommends no more than sixty minutes of screentime on school days and two hours on nonschool days.

Here are my tips for creating safety and boundaries around video game playing:

- **Make sure play happens out in the open.** Young children should play in shared spaces, not in bedrooms.
- **Avoid headsets with this age group.** Headsets may seem convenient so you don't have to hear the talking, screaming, or background music, but

when your child is starting off with video games, you'll want to hear what he's doing so you can monitor what's going on.
- **Enable ALL the parent control functions before you even give the device, app, or access to your child.** You need to set time limits for gaming, restrict which games your child is allowed to play, and control whether or not he can make in-game purchases. Make sure to set a pin so that your child cannot go in and change these settings.
- **Pay attention to the ratings of video games.** Every game has a rating. If a game is rated T for teen or M for mature, it's unlikely to be a good game for your six- to twelve-year-old! If you need more information on a specific game, you can check out online sources such as the entertainment software rating board website.
- **Have a family meeting where you talk to your child about gaming BEFORE you allow him to play games.** Talk to your child about how exciting these games are, how much people love them, and how sometimes, kids get so addicted to these games they don't even want to do other things, like go to hockey practice or play outside with friends. Explain that you're going to allow your child to have certain amount of game time each day/week: start off as conservative as possible, with thirty minutes at a time, and build up from there. Tell your child it's possible that his friends will be allowed more game time than him, but that every family is different and that "in our family, we believe in balancing screentime with other activities." The first couple of times your kid plays, be in the room, see what he's doing, or even play alongside him so you have a sense of what the game really entails.

MICROTRANSACTIONS

What parents need to know: Microtransactions are small amounts of money kids can spend within video games to buy "skins" for their characters, update a character's capabilities, or to purchase more lives within a game, among other features. Most games today, particularly those found on mobile apps, are free to download and rely on in-app purchases for revenue. Even games that consumers pay for upfront may include microtransactions. Gaming is a multibillion-dollar global market, and microtransactions account for a significant percentage of all revenue derived from video games. It follows that when you sign up for a video game for your child, you may be asked to input your credit card information. If you do this, you will need to activate the necessary settings to block and restrict your child from making microtransactions, and to set a pin so that your child can't undo these settings. And even with these restrictions in place, it's still highly likely that your child will find a way to make purchases. Individually, microtransactions may be small, but they can add up quickly, so my advice is to thoroughly check your statements on a monthly basis. Children don't always do these things in a sneaky way, sometimes they don't even realize they're being charged (as I found out the hard way when my youngest son charged $1,000 on our card playing Fortnite!).

What you should tell your children: "This video game includes in-app purchases, which are things you can buy in this game. This is how the game company makes money. When you play this game, you're going to want to spend money to make your character look or act a certain way. I've set restrictions so that you can't do that without permission."

ONLINE GAMBLING

I can imagine what you're thinking. My child is a little kid, why do I need to know about online gambling? Think again. Studies show that there is a link between video gaming and gambling, and that kids can easily progress from video games to online games like blackjack, slot machines, roulette, poker, and more. In fact, your child may already be playing games with gambling-like features. A 2020 study showed that around 40 percent of young people play video games with elements of gambling within them.

"Loot boxes" are the most common way that children are exposed to gambling within video games. Your kid may be playing what looks like an innocent, fun, age-appropriate game, but if you look closely, you'll see blinking bright-colored boxes saying "Buy, buy, buy!" And what makes this even more tempting for many kids is that what's inside the loot box is a mystery that might just be what they need to help them win the game. These boxes are irresistible to a lot of kids, and as such, they've been the subject of national and international scrutiny due to concerns that they promote compulsive or gambling-like behavior or use predatory tactics to encourage addictive consumer spending, particularly in children. In 2019, the FTC hosted a meeting in Washington, DC, on video game loot boxes and related microtransactions due to concerns that these features are priming children's brains for online gambling.[12]

Your child may also see ads or other invitations to gamble via third-party sites while playing what you thought was age-appropriate gaming. At time of writing, the platform Roblox—among the most popular games for kids under the age of twelve—has a class action lawsuit against the company due to third-party gambling sites inviting children to play blackjack, slots, roulette and other games of chance using Roblox's in-game currency, Robux. You read that right: Roblox users can start playing other gambling games *on other sites* using Robux. Another concern for parents should be online fantasy sports leagues. Sometimes kids, often boys, start betting, creating brackets, following different teams, and most parents are in the dark about how intense this can get. And so, it's time to add conversations about gambling to the list of the many talks to have with your child about screen time, especially if addiction runs in your family, or your kid shows signs of having an addictive type of personality.

What you should tell your children: "I want to talk to you about gambling and video games, because although some of the features in your games seem super fun and exciting, I want this activity to stay fun for you and not turn into a problem down the road. Gambling can be very addictive and can turn into a destructive habit—some adults get so addicted that they can't stop and lose a lot of money as a result. I don't want this to happen to you. Features like loot boxes in games are so exciting, but they are just like gambling. I know you're going to be tempted to spend your money on them. We need to train your brain not to get sucked into spending money in this way. One thing that can be helpful is to think about other things you want to save money for."

SOCIAL MEDIA

The verdict on social media is becoming clearer: it is detrimental to many and high risk for all youth. Given its damaging effects on mental health, there is a growing movement to delay the age that kids can gain access to social media.[13] In one of the first long-term studies on adolescent neural development[14] and technology use, researchers at the University of North Carolina at Chapel

Hill noted that adolescents' habitual checking of social media is linked with subsequent changes in how their brains respond to the world around them. The study, published in *JAMA Pediatrics*, reveals that adolescents' brains may become more sensitive when anticipating social rewards and punishments over time with increased social media usage. What this means is that children who grow up checking social media more often are becoming hypersensitive to feedback from their peers.

Kids who are on social media are getting too much information and material that they aren't emotionally ready for, including often unintentional exposure to images and headlines about warfare, shootings, and environmental catastrophes that are unlike anything their parents came across at this age. All it takes is signing up for a couple of apps and before you know it, your child is being bombarded with a near-constant stream of entertaining videos, snaps, memes, texts, and DMs from friends, making it harder for them to focus on offline activities or even just daydreaming and relaxing.

In the past several years, some scientists have disputed the idea that social media use itself makes kids miserable. "There's been absolutely hundreds of [social media and mental health] studies, almost all showing pretty small effects," Jeff Hancock, a behavioral psychologist at Stanford University who has conducted a meta-analysis of 226 such studies, told the *New York Times*. But I think he's missing the point. Social media isn't like rat poison, which is toxic to everyone. It's more like alcohol: an addictive substance that can enhance social situations but can also lead to dependency and depression among regular users.

This is very close to the conclusion reached by none other than Instagram. The company's internal research from 2020 found that, while most users had a positive relationship with the app, one-third of teen girls said, "Instagram made them feel worse," even though these girls "feel unable to stop themselves" from logging on. And if you don't believe a company owned by Facebook, believe a large new study from Cambridge University, in which researchers looked at 84,000 people of all ages and found that heavy social media use was strongly associated with worse mental health during two sensitive life periods, puberty, *including for girls ages eleven to thirteen*, and then again late in adolescence.

Despite some positive aspects of digital media, which include the capability to effortlessly communicate with peers, neurological consequences have been observed related to internet/gaming addiction, language development, and processing of emotional signals.[15] At the end of the day, social media makes it too easy for kids to binge on videos or content around topics like depression or weight loss, or any kind of insecurity. That is because these apps gamify the experience with the goal of making the activity (binging on posts) more engaging, motivating, and enjoyable to keep you fixated. Thanks to parent advocacy on this issue, social media platforms are finally responding by building more controls into these apps—but it's still up to you, as the parent, to implement these restrictions and to engage in an ongoing dialogue with your child about social media, its dangers, and how to stay safe.

What you should tell your children: "Social media can be fun and help you stay connected with friends, but it can also be harmful, especially for kids. Doctors say that using social media a lot can change how your brain works, making you more sensitive to what other people think about you. It can also be really distracting and make it harder to focus on learning at school. It can make you feel worried or sad, especially when you see upsetting things like bad news or scary images. Social media isn't all bad, but it's like sugar: it can be addictive and harmful if used too much."

THE ALGORITHM

An algorithm is a complex set of rules and calculations used by social media sites and streaming services to determine the content you see and the order in which you see it. This algorithm is constantly monitoring your online use to see how long you spend on certain content, whether you comment on it, like it, share it, save it, or return to it later; and then based on that, it sends you targeted posts it thinks you will like. It's programmed to show you content that tends to generate higher levels of engagement, which means that anything incendiary, outrageous, or sometimes totally untrue often ends up getting amplified or viewed millions of times. On the one hand, you can influence the algorithm by interacting with a post you like. On the other hand, the algorithm influences *you* by showing you content with the goal of harvesting data about you and making money through advertising. The downside for kids—and all of us—is that we may not get to see a full, accurate, or contextualized range of perspectives when the algorithm reinforces our existing biases and prevents us from seeing things from another viewpoint. It can also keep us stuck in a certain mindset, feeding us potentially toxic information on a topic that we might otherwise have quickly moved on from. The algorithm can be tough for adults to navigate, and even harder for a child.

What you should tell your children: "You know how on Netflix or YouTube there is a 'Recommended for you' section, which shows you other videos or shows you might like? That's because there's something called an 'algorithm' that sees what you like and shows you more of it. If you like dance videos, it will show you more dance videos, or if you like cats, you'll see more of that too. Which is so great, right? The problem is that once the algorithm learns what you like, it may not show you other information that might be interesting to you. I want you to be able to think about things from lots of different points of view, which is why we also read books and newspapers, travel to different places, and talk to people in real life to learn about how others see the world. The other problem with the algorithm is that it can keep you stuck. If you feel sad one day, you might click on a video about feeling sad, and then you will continue getting sad videos. After a while, you might start to feel overwhelmed, even if you would've otherwise moved on and started feeling happy again. If you want to, you can stop the algorithm showing you something by unfollowing, by not interacting, or by clicking 'don't show me this.' It's really important that you a take breaks from scrolling about every half hour and be with your friends in real life."

ONLINE BUSINESS MODELS

The term "attention economy" refers to the way that social media works to capture our attention and then profit from it. Social media apps are free to use, which means they are specifically engineered to keep us scrolling—using techniques such as notifications, friend suggestions, personalized feeds, "for you" page recommendations—to make money from us via advertising and data harvesting. The more time kids spend on social media, the better the platform gets at collecting data about them in order to get better at influencing their behavior, purchasing decisions, and time spent on the app. Everything your child has ever clicked on or lingered on, whether it's a post about lip oil, diet product ads, fitness influencer posts, or friends' profiles—it's all data that helps companies study and feed children more of what, at times, can be harmful for them. In other words, the attention economy is designed to be addictive: these apps keep all of us coming back for more, or staying longer in the first place, constantly pinging us to let us know that something has been posted or someone has messaged us, because that's the business model. It's how they make billions of dollars.

What you should tell your children: "I want you to understand the way social media works and how big companies profit from the time you spend on these apps. Social media is designed to grab our attention and keep us scrolling as much as possible. This is because, although social media apps are free, these companies want to make money from you in the form of ads and by gathering information about what you look at and how long you look at it. One of the ways advertising works is that it can make people feel bad about themselves, so they will buy something to try to feel better. I don't want you to feel bad about yourself just because you saw a lot of advertising, and so that's why I'm restricting the time you can spend on this app. I'm also going to turn off notifications so you're not getting constantly distracted."

DIGITAL FOOTPRINT

A digital footprint is the data you leave behind when using the internet, whether it's via websites you visit, emails you send, or information you post or submit online. Companies, websites, and even the government can use your digital footprint to learn about you. This is particularly relevant for kids. Back when you were growing up, you made mistakes, said things you wished you could take back, or had things happen that were embarrassing. The difference between now and then is that your child is going through these same developmental phases while being constantly documented, all of which creates a permanent digital record. Before a child even turns eighteen, he's going to have a massive online footprint that may include embarrassing photos, videos, online searches, and more. This doesn't give children a lot of leeway for making the kinds of mistakes that are typical of growing up. And while some apps like Snapchat may claim that posts are deleted, your child should know that, in fact, those images still live on in the cloud. Instead of thinking "My kid is too young to have a digital footprint, I don't have to deal with this," you should think, "My child is going to have a digital footprint, and now's the time to start getting educated on how to guide him about this."

What you should tell your children: "Your digital footprint is what's created anytime you click anything online; when you put something in a search engine, send a text or email, post a photo, or make a comment. Whatever you put online is out there and never really goes away: it's even more lasting than a tattoo. It could be shared by someone else, and suddenly hundreds or even thousands of people might see it. Even if an app says that your pictures, video or message is going to be deleted, it will still live in the cloud or on someone else's phone. You should never post photos of yourself doing things that can get you into trouble. These photos could be seen years into the future when you're trying to get into college or get a job and they could be held against you. You can have a positive digital footprint by putting things online that reflect your kindness, hard work, and achievements. If someone posts a photo of you and tags you in a photo that you don't want your name attached to, you can remove the tag or hide the post from your profile."

INFLUENCER CULTURE

Social media influencers are people who have large followings online. They make money or get free products from brands who compensate them to use their products and post about them. A recent survey revealed that more than half of Gen Z kids want to be influencers, which tells you a lot about how powerful these figures have become in our culture. Being an influencer is the top career aspiration of teens today. Once your child is on social media, he's unknowingly entering a world of influence, in which he will be the target of people who want to sell him things. It's a world that's largely unknown to parents, because when we go into our social media feeds, we see entirely different content. If your child follows influencers online, he will likely know a lot about them: everything from their pets' name to their favorite drink at Starbucks, and their relationship issues. Influencers usually use filters and lighting to make themselves look more attractive, and they may have had cosmetic procedures to look the way they do, creating unrealistic beauty and body standards, and feeding into young people's feelings of insecurity or lack of self-worth.

What you should tell your children: "I know you look up to the people you see online, and you might feel like they are your friend, or a cool big sister or brother. But what you need to understand is that influencers are paid to use and then sell certain brands and products. They may use filters and lighting to make themselves or the product look better. They will tell you they are truly in love with a product that they're using, but we may never know whether they really are or not—as they're being paid to tell us that. They work hard at gaining your trust, but I want you to know an influencer is not your friend: an influencer is being paid to make a commercial. Just because they look a certain way, or wear certain things, that doesn't mean you have to try to look that way too. When deciding to follow someone, you can ask yourself how you feel when you see a post from that person. If seeing a post doesn't make you feel good—unfollow them! And if someone who comments on your posts makes you feel bad about yourself, block them."

BEAUTY CULTURE

Prior to social media, the biggest influences on how we looked and felt about ourselves were movies, magazines, and TV shows. Today, across the board, social media sets the standards. The young women dominating social media feeds conform to an almost universal version of "beauty": they have smooth, and dewy skin, high cheekbones, almond-shaped eyes, long lashes, a small nose and full lips, bright white teeth, and long, straight, often lightened hair. In terms of body types, they're slender, with a narrow waist, curves, and an athletic, but not too muscular, physique. They're constantly trying on new outfits or beauty products and showing them off to their followers. For boys, the young men on social media have six-pack abs, square jaws, muscular shoulders, chests, and arms, with low body fat. These young male influencers are likely selling you fitness plans, skin care products, and clothing. And if you don't happen to have an Instagram-perfect face or hair or body, there are filters on social media to help you achieve that flawless skin, make you thinner, give you a squarer jaw, or whatever your heart desires—and you can always buy the clothing and products, which the influencers in your feed are being paid to advertise to you. If your child is suddenly asking for expensive hair and cosmetic products, new clothes, or fitness or diet plans, you'll know why.

Kids don't magically wake up one morning and decide they need these things. If your child starts following and interacting with certain influencers, eventually he loses free will to explore other types of content. He'll be fed similar videos over and over until he begins to believe this must be the only way to look. Kids' feeds end up dominated by images of generically "beautiful" and skinny young women and men, and these images, in turn, have been linked to low self-esteem, less confidence, body image problems, eating disorders, and even kids wanting to get plastic surgery to conform to what they're seeing online. The concentration of similar and consistent messages around beauty ideals can overwhelm a child's vulnerabilities and insecurities. Ten- to fourteen-year-old girls are particularly susceptible to the social validation effects of social media related to beauty and identity, which is why I suggest starting conversations around beauty culture with your child by or around age ten. Research shows that four out of five girls would like their parents to talk to them about how to manage toxic beauty advice on social media.[16] Although girls are most affected, research shows that boys are also being sucked in by these kinds of idealized images, so it's important to talk to your boys too.

What you should tell girls: "As you're starting to go online more, and watching more videos, you're going to see videos of girls showing you how they put their makeup on, or what clothes they buy, or which hair products they use. I want you to know that these people are paid to look a certain way, that they use filters, lighting and makeup to look the way they do. This can make us feel like we have to look that same way to be liked by other people. But the truth is, everyone is unique and beautiful in their own way, and what's most important is how we feel about ourselves on the inside. It's okay to have fun with makeup and express your style, but it's also important to remember that true beauty comes from being kind, confident, and authentic."

What you should tell boys: "Now that you're going online, you might see images of boys and young men who look a certain way. The boys may have a certain hairstyle, six-pack abs, they may have a lot of muscles. You may feel like you need to look that way too. But you have to remember: the people in those videos are using lighting and filters to highlight the parts of their bodies they want you to see. They're being paid by companies to sell you products. They're not your friends. The way you look doesn't define who you are: who you are is defined by how kind you are and how you treat others."

Digital Detox

A digital detox is when you take a break from using digital devices like smartphones and social media.[17] It's a way to disconnect from screens and spend more time doing other things like playing and hanging out with friends and family. This break can help you and/or your child feel less stressed, sleep better, and improve your overall well-being. It does this by reducing the level of cortisol running through your body and giving it the ability to relax. Families tell me that when they implement a digital detox it gives kids a glimpse of what life was like before screens.

How do you know when your kid may need a detox?

- Your child feels the need to check his phone constantly or be on a video game whenever he can.
- He can't concentrate unless he checks his device often. He may need the laptop to do homework but can't help wandering off to do other things while using it.
- He feels that he's missing out on something if he's not checking his phone—aka FOMO (fear of missing out).
- After spending time on a screen, he has a hard time transitioning off without a noticeable mood swing.
- If he can't be on his device, or it gets taken away, it feels stressful and puts him in a bad mood.
- He stays up late watching something or playing a game, which is causing him to go to bed later.
- He begins comparing himself to others on social media and feels bad about himself.
- He skips hanging out with people in person because he would rather be home playing a video game.

This isn't an official checklist; it's based on my experience as a psychologist and mom. If you answered yes to even one of these, it is a yellow flag. If you answered yes to two or more that is a red flag. The sooner you can introduce detoxes, the easier a kid will accept that too much of a good thing is not good for him. Breaks are good. They can vary in length from a weekend to a week, to a whole vacation, to a summer! And when it's done, ask your kid how that felt, what he noticed. You can teach him that it's okay to admit that it was kind of nice to do other things, that he will still get a screen back, but that balance is what we are striving for.

Looking Ahead

Looking ahead, you need to understand that once your child becomes a teenager, most of his social life will be online. Pregnancies, vehicle deaths, and in-person bullying are down partly because teenagers *are spending more time by themselves and less time together*. Before you know it, kids turn into tweens and teens who will start using curse words, making inappropriate jokes, and looking up sex. Group chats are the new cliques, and kids don't use text, they only communicate via Snapchat. They get one another's snaps rather than their phone numbers. They spend hours a day video chatting, sending pictures of themselves or their walls to one another, and each pose, ceiling, floor, or half face actually means something. They have a visual language and three to five letter codes that also hold a lot of power. They have rank orders of best friends according to how much they communicate, and they connect with teens far and wide, not just their high school, due to these apps making friend suggestions. Things that parents may think mean something, like a crush started following them, may not actually mean anything at all. Because a follow can mean just that, a simple click because a code told them to. And so, if in the next few years, you are lost and don't understand what most of this means, just ask them!

In a Nutshell

- Create screen-free zones in your home and don't let kids sleep with screens.
- Be a good digital role model.

- Set clear boundaries and stick to them.
- Learn to use the parental controls on every device, browser, and app your child uses.
- Talk about digital literacy with your child.
- Monitor your child's activity online.
- Show an interest in your child's online world.
- Don't give your child a screen when he's upset or to distract him.
- Collaborate with other parents and your child's school to set healthy expectations around screen use.
- "Wait Until 8th" to give your child a phone and until high school for social media.
- If you do give your child a phone at this age, make him sign a phone contract.
- Pay attention to the ratings of games.
- Talk about online gambling with your child.
- Give your child real books to read.
- Value offline, unstructured play, particularly outside.
- Do a regular digital detox with your child.

CHAPTER 9

Substances

> I've gotten away with a lot in my life. The older you get the more you realize you're not getting away with it, it's taking its toll somewhere. So, you try not to put yourself in those situations. Part of the mysterious process called growing up. Some people do that better than others.
>
> —Jon Hamm

This is a book about the overlap between middle childhood and puberty, so we shouldn't have to worry too much about substance use, right?

Meet Emilia, who revealed to me my own naivete around this issue. Emilia was a straight-A student who came out of fifth grade as a well-liked good athlete whose only apparent issue was that she could be a people pleaser. She was described by teachers and neighbors as a delight to be around, and the last child anyone would worry about vaping, doing drugs, drinking alcohol, or getting into trouble.

I began seeing Emilia when she was in the middle of sixth grade because her mother, Celeste, thought she seemed anxious and not herself. After Celeste tried to get her daughter to tell her what was going on—but didn't get anywhere—she decided to reach out for help. When I met Emilia, she was polite, articulate, and seemingly open. As she started to trust me, she disclosed that she had started cutting herself sometimes at night in her room and that she had feelings of low self-worth. She was restricting food and becoming more secretive in other subtle ways, like skipping lunch at school while keeping the money she was given.

Over the course of our first few months together, I felt we were headed in a positive direction, given that Emilia reported to me the cutting was reduced to an occasional level and her parents were now aware and checking her, while making sure she ate breakfast and dinner. We established a positive rapport during the winter and spring of her sixth-grade year. We had once a month of family therapy sessions and those also seemed to improve communication and help the parents in supporting Emilia. Her mom and dad realized that running their other two kids around to a different school in the morning and then to after-school activities—plus working two jobs—left the family feeling disjointed. They'd never had to worry about Emilia before as she was responsible and independent; she rode her bike or walked to school and maintained good grades. It was easy to see how things could slip through the cracks, and we all felt as if a new safety net was in place for Emilia.

Imagine my disbelief when, during the last two weeks of the school year, Emilia's parents learned that their twelve-year-old honor student had not only tried marijuana but had progressed to being a "drug plug" (slang for the middleman in a drug deal). When her school got wind that vape pens with weed had been found on campus, an investigation ensued. Eventually, Emilia's name was mentioned as being involved and school administrators were told that she owed some eighth graders some money for vapes they had given her money for, but she hadn't delivered them.

Like Emilia's parents, you might also assume you don't have to think about or worry about drugs and alcohol until maybe high school. And even then that it will be innocent, a fifteen-year-old trying a little weed or some alcohol, part of experimenting as a teenager—many parents remember doing the same at that age. The problem is that a lot has changed since we were that age. Legalization of marijuana and the easier availability of more powerful opioids are widening kids' exposure to substances that can be abused. You likely grew up with (mainly ineffective) drug-use prevention programs such as Scared Straight and D.A.R.E., but today, we don't have new and proven strategies for keeping our kids safe. Earlier puberty is actually a risk factor for substance abuse. Almost 11 percent of eighth graders reported using illicit substances in 2023.

And so middle childhood *is* the time to teach kids about alcohol, marijuana, vaping, and even opioids—which they will likely be exposed to or even try sooner than you think. Emilia was warned that she would meet people in her new, large inner-city public middle school who vaped in bathrooms and used drugs. In fifth grade she had participated in a substance-use prevention program. She came home and told her parents things she learned and the games they played and small-group conversations they had. The parents thought this was great—she seemed educated and low risk, so they weren't worried. Yet despite being told about the dangers, this smart and sweet kid fell victim to peer pressure.

A month before sixth grade started, Emilia had met a group of thirteen- and fourteen-year-old kids, rising eighth graders at her soon-to-be-school, at the park near her house. At first, she said that when offered marijuana she said "no," she felt uncomfortable, but stayed while they did it, and no one pressured her. She told her friend it didn't seem so scary, that the kids smoking were laughing and acting pretty fine. When she met up with them the next week, this time with a friend in tow, she said she felt like she couldn't say no. Emilia's friend told her she would do it first so she could see that she would be okay, and the other kids told her to just try one hit, that no one would even know, and it wouldn't be a big deal. Emilia recounted the story while crying. She was hard on herself, saying she should have known better, that it wasn't even that much peer pressure, and that she was mad at herself for not being able to say no again.

Emilia started watching TikTok videos about how "weed isn't bad for you" and talking to other kids who agreed. In fact, she was buying into the notion that—because recreational marijuana use had been legal in Colorado for about five years at that point, with a dispensary on almost every corner, and the smell of weed anywhere you go—it couldn't be that bad. She then started getting fed videos by social media algorithms about how prescription pills for anxiety or pain are worse than THC (tetrahydrocannabinol, the psychoactive compound found in marijuana) and if you're struggling with mental issues, it's better to smoke weed than to take psychiatric medications. According to these videos, drug companies are "out to make money," and the government "just wants to control people."

It's easy to understand how kids today are vulnerable to these types of messages. There's widespread acceptance of CBD products (containing cannabidiol that's derived from cannabis but without THC) for almost anything you can imagine, including for pets. At the time of this writing, cannabis is recreationally legal and available in twenty-four states where more than half of Americans live. There is a normalization of use all around, especially in the music some tweens and most teens listen to, making it even more likely children will be exposed to and may consume marijuana products, possibly in the form of edibles, such as gummies, cookies, or brownies. There are also infused lotions, tinctures, drinks, and sprays in addition to inhaling it through joints, bongs, and vapes.

Children experiencing earlier puberty, combined with conditions like ADHD, anxiety, or depression, face unique challenges that increase their risk of turning to substances as a coping mechanism. Earlier puberty can cause self-consciousness, a feeling of growing up faster, being treated older, and social pressures. A condition such as ADHD can lead to impulsivity, challenges with keeping friends, and a propensity toward being a class-clown type for attention. As kids get older and that wears off, they can more easily give into impulses for higher risk behavior than other kids their age. Anxiety and depression may drive adolescents to self-medicate with substances to manage overwhelming emotions, a sense of restlessness, and social isolation. These factors, coupled with a lack of effective coping strategies and potentially higher vulnerability to peer pressure, heighten the risk of substance use.

As your child approaches the end of elementary school and begins middle school, you will need to make a habit of talking to her regularly about drugs, alcohol, and tobacco in a way that's appropriate to her level of understanding and age. Make your views on the subject clear and repeat them often. If you don't approve of smoking or drinking, be sure your child knows this and the reasons for your beliefs. Your child needs to understand that under no circumstances is drug use acceptable and that there are no safe street drugs. Be prepared to answer personal questions—at some point kids may ask you when you first drank or if you have ever tried drugs; think about what you will say. Your child is looking to you to lead the way on these issues, and it's important to make sure you are the most powerful voice on this issue—not peers.

Marijuana

In 2014, Colorado, my home state, became the first state to pass a law making the recreational use of marijuana legal. As a result, we have been on the forefront of what has since been replicated throughout the country. Soon after the law went into effect, I was invited on Katie Couric's talk show, where she asked me if I thought that marijuana was a gateway drug. I said that I think marijuana is a gateway drug to high-risk behavior. At the time, there were people who questioned that statement—but over a decade later I stand by it. If a kid is willing to smoke, vape, or eat/drink one drug, they are more likely to smoke, vape, or eat/drink another drug. Cannabis use is associated with heavy drinking and alcohol use disorders. Cannabis dependence doubles the risk for long-term continual alcohol-related problems.[1]

After the law changed, it didn't take long for the referral calls to start for kids who had eaten too many edibles and ended up in the ER, or from middle schools who wanted me to present to their students on this topic, or for requests from news outlets to comment on stories of toddlers accidentally consuming edibles. I also noticed that the teens in my center were reporting increased use and access. They started debating me on the drug's healing properties and the fact that cannabis was around Before Christ (BC) and on and on. I didn't need to wait for facts, figures, and randomized data to confirm what I feared would happen after legalization: I witnessed it firsthand, and I knew it was bad for kids. I started including marijuana education for middle schoolers who I treated alongside their families. Given the changes in marijuana since we were teenagers, most parents aren't up-to-date with what to say, especially for kids under the age of thirteen.

Due to legalization of marijuana and its prevalence in our culture, weed is everywhere these days. Unlike when I was a child, kids today are inundated with weed references everywhere from clothing to shows, and on social media. It is no wonder that teenage marijuana use is at its highest level in thirty years.

To complicate matters further, the marijuana available today is much more potent than it was in previous generations—and it comes in new packaging that's terrifyingly attractive to kids. Levels of THC have been steadily rising in marijuana since the 1970s. Just how much stronger is today's cannabis? There is no way to comprehensively assess all types of marijuana currently available either legally or illegally around the world. But the data we do have suggest that today's drug is much stronger than the weed of even a few years ago, let alone several decades prior. In the 1990s, the average THC content in marijuana was typically around 3 to 4 percent. By the mid- to late 2000s, it became increasingly common for marijuana strains to have THC levels exceeding 15 percent, with some high-potency strains reaching levels of 20 percent or higher. The National Institute on Drug Abuse through the University of Mississippi collects data on THC potency. The data show a clear trend: over the last fifty years, the average amount of THC in cannabis—the plant's main psychoactive component—has increased more than tenfold.[2] And with easy access in many states to edibles, you can imagine how problematic this is for children and teens.

Accordingly, ER visits for children sick from marijuana have surged—with the biggest jump among kids under age eleven, with a more than 200 percent increase, according to the CDC. There's a common misconception that marijuana is harmless, which makes kids more open to trying it.[3] In fact, there are serious risks involved in smoking or consuming marijuana at young ages while the brain is still developing. Besides the fact that it will impair your judgment and possibly make you do something dangerous, studies show that regular cannabis use in adolescence can affect attention, memory, learning, and executive function.[4]

Another significant risk these days is fentanyl-laced marijuana. This is marijuana contaminated with fentanyl, a potent synthetic opioid that's added to enhance the immediate effects of marijuana and/or to increase profits by adding weight to the product. The combination of fentanyl and marijuana is particularly hazardous and often goes undetected, posing a significant risk of overdose and potentially fatal consequences. This risk is exacerbated for individuals without prior exposure to fentanyl, who lack tolerance to this powerful substance, making even small amounts extremely dangerous and fatal. It seems as if every week there's another article of a young person who has died from an accidental fentanyl death, completely unaware that the drug was present in what they were using.

The way people consume cannabis has also been shifting. The edibles, vapes, and other forms that have been growing in popularity are much easier to pack with THC. Some concentrates have THC levels of up to 90 percent, including hash oil, THC distillate, cannabis wax, shatter, and live resin. However, due to their high THC content, they can also pose greater risks of overconsumption and adverse effects. The teens I work with who admit to using marijuana call it "greening out," when they essentially overdose on marijuana. At least they now know that overdosing on marijuana is a real thing; years ago kids didn't believe that was possible.

I know there are big opinions on both sides of this issue among parents, so I say that even if you are a user yourself, or don't believe there is anything wrong with marijuana use, or that it's better than alcohol, please consider three major factors when it comes to keeping your kids safe in today's ever-changing world: the increased potency, the vulnerability of the developing brain until age twenty-five, and the prevalence of fentanyl-laced marijuana.

In 2024, Colorado decriminalized personal use and cultivation of psilocybin mushrooms for people age twenty-one and older, with regulated therapy centers expected to open in 2025, providing supervised access to these substances for healing purposes. There are strong cases to be made about the medicinal properties of CBD in marijuana and of psilocybin mushroom microdosing for mental health issues like PTSD and depression. However, my unique concern is for the impact this will likely have on children, including easier access for experimentation, accidental consumption by younger children who may find it in their home, and the normalization of using psychedelics by teens seeking out the experience of hallucinating while their brain is still developing. Simply put, I am concerned it will result in an increase in teens tripping out on "magic" mushrooms, experiencing "bad trips," and mixing psilocybin with prescribed psychiatric medications, which can cause unpredictable psychological reactions, all while their brains are still very much under development.

HOW TO TALK TO YOUR CHILD ABOUT MARIJUANA USE

Before you start, ask your child what she knows about this topic—you can say something like "What have you heard about drugs?" as an opening statement. Then you can carefully cover each of these topics:

- **What it is:** Explain to your child that marijuana is a plant containing chemicals that can affect the brain and body when consumed in any way. Keep the explanation simple and include the known potential risks and dangers such as *impaired judgment* (your friend tells you that jumping off roofs into pools is fun: off marijuana you think that sounds dangerous, on marijuana you think that's funny); *coordination* (no, you can't drive while high); and *memory* (yes, you really do lose IQ points if you smoke marijuana while the brain is developing). If it is legal in your state, this conversation may take on a longer form—that's okay, just keep it simple, factual, and straightforward.

- **The laws:** Depending on the laws in your area, you may need to discuss the legal status of marijuana and explain that it is illegal for children to use or possess marijuana. In the US, marijuana is illegal under the federal Controlled Substances Act, but most of the country has legalized some form of medical marijuana, and half of the country's states have legalized marijuana for recreational use by people over the age of twenty-one. Help your child understand the consequences of breaking the law and the importance of following rules. Mental illness and marijuana don't mix: if there is a preexisting mental health condition in your family or child, marijuana can exacerbate those symptoms. Make sure your child is aware of this. In the past couple of years, marijuana-induced psychosis has become a serious issue in emergency room departments. More potent cannabis and more frequent use are contributing to higher rates of psychosis, especially in young people.[5]
- **Peer pressure:** Talk to your kid about peer pressure and how to resist pressure from friends or classmates to try marijuana or other drugs. Teach her strategies for saying no assertively, teach her critical thinking skills and decision-making strategies, and use role-playing as a way to practice, even if she thinks it's silly. (You can do this with any topic, not just drugs.) Teaching your child to set and maintain boundaries is also very helpful when you're guiding her to resist peer pressure. Again, practice with lower risk issues, like a friend pressuring her to sneak the iPad so they can text at night. And last, talk about good friendship qualities. Speak about things like trust, integrity, inclusivity, and how if a friend pressures you to do something you aren't comfortable with you need to take a break from that friend. At this age, children need clear guidance on resisting pressure to do something they don't want to do.
- **Healthy choices:** Emphasize the importance of making healthy choices and taking care of your brain and body. Encourage your child to focus on activities and hobbies that promote physical and mental well-being, such as sports, creative pursuits, and spending time with family and friends. Point out the importance of making healthy choices, such as not eating too much sugar, getting quality sleep, wearing a helmet—and, eventually, not doing drugs.

Alcohol

Leah and Joel were referred to me by their couple's counselor for a parenting consultation. These are often some of my most effective sessions, because they are typically with parents who are highly motivated and want to come in for a few sessions to get educated and feel empowered about a certain issue.

In our sessions, both Leah and Joel shared that they were both adult children of alcoholics (ACOAs as they're sometimes referred to) and they wanted to explore how—or if—to share this with their boys, who were nine and eleven at the time. Joel explained that he was able to drink socially and occasionally but had not experienced any misuse or dependence. Leah on the other hand felt like her drinking had started to escalate after she had her second son. She said that she went from being a casual drinker—who felt like she escaped the grip of alcoholism she'd seen in her dad and grandfather—to all of a sudden drinking daily in the late afternoon, looking forward to two or three glasses of wine, and craving a drink at times of stress. This scared her, and after about six months led to her attending AA and ACOA meetings and committing to a life of sobriety.

Now their son was about to start middle school, they felt they needed to be clear on what they wanted to say to him on the topic of alcohol. Did they want to say alcohol is a disease that runs in their family and therefore he should completely be abstinent? Did they want to say that casual use was okay? Did they want to have a relaxed attitude toward alcohol and to not steer their son toward it when he's a rebellious teenager? They had listened to people's thoughts in groups, they had read some about it, but they still wanted to really talk this through.

One of the issues we spent some time on was their "attitude" toward alcohol. I shared with them that children whose parents have *less* restrictive attitudes toward their child's alcohol use were more likely to start drinking than their peers whose parents were *more* restrictive. A permissive, either pro-alcohol or alcohol-neutral home, can lead to the normalization of drinking and a familial blindness to the risks and harms associated with alcohol use at any level. Kids raised by parents with a permissive, less restrictive attitude toward alcohol also drank and got drunk more frequently. This is believed to be based, in part, on the *perception* of their parents' attitudes. It could be that those kids' perceptions are skewed toward thinking (but not knowing for sure) that their parents have more lenient attitudes. A compelling thought around this is that this could be because their parents haven't expressed their attitudes in a way that the children really understand. In other words, parents need to be clear about the message they want their children to hear. And if you are anything like Leah or Joel, you may realize you need to create some time and space to gain clarity on your views before talking to your child in direct terms.[6]

Alcohol is the most widely used substance among America's youth and it can cause enormous health and safety risks, with early-onset use (under the age of ten) associated with later life dependency, ill health, and poor social functioning.[7] Nonetheless, a University of Cambridge study found that 8 percent of kids have been drunk by the age of thirteen, and other studies show that it's the leading contributor to the burden of disease among youth. The changes alcohol causes in the developing brain can result in children experiencing alcohol as more rewarding as they grow older. Children who begin drinking by age thirteen have a 45 percent chance of becoming alcohol dependent later in life. That's a four times greater chance than children who do not.[8] While adolescence is an important developmental period characterized by a rapid increase of substance experimentation and use, we know that alcohol use by younger children occurs, is under-researched, and its impact is detrimental.

Many parents believe that children aged six to twelve are too young to understand alcohol and its role in our lives. In fact, children as young as *two years old* are aware of alcohol and are able to tell by looking at the drink, whether an adult is drinking an alcoholic or nonalcoholic drink. Children as young as four years old can begin to comprehend what type of alcohol use is normal in their family and they create expectations related to its use. Many parents assume their children don't notice their drinking, especially when they're young, so the negative impacts caused are often unintentional on the part of parents. Kids start to form their own beliefs and assumptions about alcohol based on their observations and experiences typically beginning with their parents' use.

But here's some *relatively* good news: underage drinking is on the decline. One study found that past-month consumption among eighth graders had decreased 41 percent over ten years, reaching a record low 6 percent. Another study found that fewer than 2 percent of kids aged twelve to thirteen reported drinking the previous month. But that doesn't mean your child won't be affected. Looking ahead, about 10 percent of twelve-year-olds say they have tried alcohol, but by age fifteen, that number jumps to 50 percent. Additionally, by the time they are seniors, almost 70 percent of high school students will have tried alcohol.

So when should you talk to your child about this important issue? The research suggests that parents should start talking about drinking and other substance use when children are between ages five and seven and that you keep the discussion going from there.

When talking to your child, keep in mind that peer pressure is considered to be the most influential factor on a young person's decision to drink alcohol. This important stage of adolescence is all about identity and fitting in; talking to your child about what is common, what may happen, and providing them with alternatives to drinking can be an effective way to either prevent or delay alcohol use. Talking with your child at a young age is especially important if family members have alcohol or drug problems. Children with a family history of substance abuse are more likely to become substance abusers.

HOW TO TALK TO YOUR CHILD ABOUT ALCOHOL

- Look for teachable moments. For example, if you drink wine with dinner, talk about why you drink, why children don't drink, and what it means to drink responsibly. Or if your child is watching TV and a beer commercial comes on, discuss the fact that although the people in the commercial appear to be having a good time, drinking too much alcohol can cause you to make bad decisions.
- Make it clear that you disapprove of alcohol use for kids under the age of twenty-one. Research suggests that children are less likely to drink alcohol when their parents make it clear that they do not agree with it.
- Talk about the connection between feeling stressed and using substances. Explain that there are other ways to help when you feel that way and using substances to cope is never a good idea. Avoid making statements around your kid like "I need a whole bottle of wine right now!" or "Oh, I needed that" after having a beer. Don't send your child the message that alcohol is a solution to stress. Children are aware of parental motivations for drink-

ing, so if you show them that you drink to release the stress of the day, they will hear that message loud and clear.
- Model moderation. Deliberately drink only a small amount of alcohol, or nothing at all, around your children at home.

Remember, research indicates that alcohol use during the teenage years can interfere with normal adolescent brain development and increase the risk of developing alcohol use disorder. In addition, underage drinking contributes to a range of acute consequences, such as injuries, sexual assaults, alcohol overdoses, and death—including those from car accidents. The sooner you talk to your child about alcohol and other drugs, the greater chance you have of influencing her decisions around drinking and substance use in times when you aren't around and she needs to make her own choices.[9] You want your thoughts and talks to be like a little birdie in her head.

Nicotine

Renee and Tessa, mothers of a son about to enter eighth grade, never suspected he was vaping. They felt they had been clear about the fact that this was dangerous for his health and had talked to him about this issue at length after attending an info night at his school in sixth grade. But when Renee went through Julian's phone and found multiple "saved in chat" videos on Snapchat where her son was blowing smoke around like a pro—right in his bedroom, with family downstairs, in the daylight—they realized they'd assumed wrong. Both parents confronted Julian, demanding he hand over the vape, then searching his entire room to find the vape. Eventually, Julian gave it up (who knows if there were more): he had it hidden in his school backpack mixed in with his markers, pencils, and pens. "Even if we looked, we never would have spotted it," Renee pointed out. "It looked like a pen." Their son eventually admitted he was vaping in the school bathroom, at friends' houses, and at home. What had started off as something he felt pressured to do at school became something he then felt pressured to do before baseball practice, then cravings started, and he did it at home—sometimes snapping images of the vape smoke to friends.

In 2018, US Surgeon General Jerome Adams officially declared e-cigarette (vape) use among youth an "epidemic" after a dramatic and sharp rise in vape use was tracked in teens. A 2019 study found that 17.6 percent of eighth graders had vaped in the previous year. Studies have also found that kids who smoke e-cigarettes are more likely to smoke regular cigarettes when they become older and can legally purchase them.[10] E-cigarettes or vapes are devices that heat a liquid into an aerosol the user inhales; the liquids come in various flavors, which are particularly appealing to teens. Brands like JUUL have been specifically noted for their high nicotine content and sleek, easily concealable designs that attract adolescents (JUUL was banned in 2022 but it seems like every year there are new brands coming onto the market.)

E-cigarettes are hooking a new generation on nicotine—putting millions of kids at risk and threatening decades of progress in reducing youth tobacco use. It's a nationwide crisis of youth addiction, fueled by thousands of kid-friendly flavors and massive doses of nicotine. (Sometimes kids say they vape the nicotine-free options, though it is difficult to tell if this is really the case.) E-cigarettes are the most commonly used tobacco product among youth in the US and nicotine remains the most commonly used vaping substance for this group. Data suggest vaping nicotine may introduce the substance to youth who would otherwise not have smoked cigarettes or used nicotine through another tobacco product.

So, what's driving this vaping trend? When I gave a talk at a private middle and high school years ago, before the pandemic, I spoke with teens who had vaped, and those who had never vaped before. Both groups spoke about the popularity and acceptance among their peers to vape, but not to smoke cigarettes. The research on teen vaping points to peer influence (having peers who use tobacco) as one of the most common drivers of teen e-cigarette use. It is important to point out that *influence*, even more so than pressure, is noted by adolescents as a main driver. Social acceptance (popularity, fitting in) plays a role in curiosity and interest in vaping. Exposure to e-cigarette marketing and advertising is also associated with an openness to experimenting with e-cigarettes. The most common source for a vape is a friend, followed by a family member. A quarter of youth live with someone who uses e-cigarettes, which plays a role: a third of youth who live with an e-cigarette user reported receiving or buying e-cigarettes from a family member, a higher proportion compared to those not living with an e-cigarette user.[11]

According to industry standards, a single milliliter of vape juice typically provides roughly one hundred puffs. This means that one milliliter of vape juice is approximately equivalent to five packs of cigarettes. So, in the palm of a person's hand, in a small vial, there are five packs of cigarettes. There are so many concerns about this, but for me thinking about children in middle childhood, I think about the critical role of prevention and—if you can't prevent it—how important it is to delay it. **Children are more susceptible to addiction than adults,** and the earlier a person is exposed to nicotine the more likely they are to be addicted throughout their lifetime.[12] Addiction takes place in the limbic system—the reward center of the brain—which makes teens uniquely vulnerable to early substance use becoming problematic.

The ages of six through twelve truly represent a window of opportunity to prevent or at least delay exposure to substances to prevent lifelong use. And when it comes to vaping, the pressure that kids feel to try it and continue to use it at parties and in school bathrooms is a lot for an impressionable preteen or teen. The conversations you have now, being sure to include the respiratory health risks—as well as the boundary setting, decision-making, and critical thinking skills you're teaching your kid in middle childhood—can be effective to prevention.

NICOTINE POUCHES

Nicotine pouches are a type of oral, smokeless tobacco-free product. They are small bags or pouches containing nicotine that's extracted from the tobacco plant, along with other ingredients such as flavorings and sweeteners. These pouches are placed between the upper lip and gum, where the nicotine is absorbed through the mucous membranes of the mouth.

Nicotine pouches do not contain tobacco leaf; instead, they use a tobacco-derived nicotine extract combined with fillers like cellulose. They're an ideal way for young people to consume nicotine because they don't produce smoke or require spitting, and they come in various flavors and strengths.

Nicotine pouches are marketed as an alternative to smoking and vaping and as a harm-reduction option for smokers looking to quit or limit their tobacco use. However, they still contain nicotine, and the health risks are being researched. A popular brand, ZYN, is very popular with young people with social media "ZYNfluencers," who are typically young, attractive adults who look like college kids. These people promote that ZYN helps them lose weight and gives them energy, among other claims. ZYN is being consumed by youth, and parents are usually totally in the dark about this. It also comes in flavors like citrus and mint, once again highly appealing to younger people. Making sure that your middle schooler is aware that you know what this is before high school is the way to go.

Here are some nicotine facts to share with your kids. Before you start, ask your child what she knows about the topic. Then say the following:

- Nicotine can lead to anxiety. If you start to consume nicotine and then decide you want to stop, your body can go into what is called "withdrawal" and you can be irritable, have mood swings, have a hard time focusing, and experience trouble sleeping.
- Nicotine is linked to an increased risk of cancer. Although the long-term health effects of e-cigarettes are not yet fully understood, studies show vaping is not a safe or healthy alternative to smoking. Vaping can increase the risk of lung cancer due to the dangerous chemicals that are in the liquid.
- If you are around someone who is smoking, you should get out of that space. Secondhand smoke can cause heart disease or cancer, even if you never smoked a single cigarette.
- Consuming nicotine while your body is still developing impacts the healthy development of your brain, affecting learning, memory, attention, mood, and impulse control.

Looking Ahead

As your child grows well into the teenage years, you'll need to shift the conversation around substances to focus on harm reduction. Simply put, harm reduction means that you accept that your child *may* drink at parties or *may* try weed, and therefore you need to talk about moderation and safety planning such as not getting behind the wheel with anyone who has been drinking or using drugs. This may include talking to kids with preexisting mental health conditions or a family history of addiction and helping them understand their increased risk of depression, anxiety, mania, hallucinations, and addiction if they use drugs. The alternative to harm reduction is to rely on school policy, your kid's strong will, public awareness campaigns, or denial that your kid won't ever try alcohol or drugs. I get it—none of us want to think about our precious child engaging in high-risk behaviors when they're a teen, it's scary. But it is the reality.

In a Nutshell

- Start to talk to your child earlier than you may want to about substances, and definitely by the end of elementary school.
- Make sure your child understands that substances are harmful for developing brains and bodies and that her brain will continue to develop until she's twenty-five.
- Keep an eye on your child for any behavior that might indicate that drug, alcohol, or vape use is going on.
- Lead the way on educating your kid. Don't solely rely on programs at school or public health campaigns.
- Talk to your child about peer pressure and how to stand up to it.
- Model abstinence or moderation for your child and talk to her about why you do this.
- Keep your child involved in activities that are healthy mentally and physically.
- Be realistic about the risk that your child may engage in substance use as they enter high school and do what you can now to prevent or reduce harm.

Epilogue

Throughout the course of this book, I've introduced you to the most essential factors in raising a happy, healthy, and confident six- to twelve-year-old in this modern age. Although each child is uniquely different, I hope that this book has inspired you to think more deeply about these crucial years of middle childhood. My goal in writing about this phase has been to help you build a strong parent-child relationship based on psychological safety and open communication, enabling your child to navigate the challenges of middle childhood and the teen years with confidence, resilience, competence, and security. And I want *you* to also feel empowered as you find your way through the challenges you will likely face as a parent with a child this age. I want you to lean in to your greater understanding of your child's development, so that you can support your child's emotional and psychological well-being today and in the future. In every decision you make about your child, I want you to think to yourself, "Will this help my child feel more industrious? If I allow my child to do this, or, better yet, if I hold my child back from doing this, what might my child learn? Will he or she feel more accomplished, competent, and secure?"

As I wrote the scripts included in this book—re-creating the potentially awkward or difficult conversations that you will hopefully have around puberty, sexuality, and relationships in an open and nonjudgmental way going forward—I pictured the many kids, including my own, that I have sat across from having the same conversations. I'm grateful to them for opening up and trusting me so that I could share with you what has worked for us, them, and their families. As we come to the end of this book, I want to remind you that no parent or child is ever truly alone in their journey, and that many of the joys and challenges you may currently be facing are the same ones experienced by your neighbors and friends—many of whom may not want to talk about these topics until someone else is vulnerable enough to share their own experiences first. I hope that now that you have read this book, you will feel more open and curious about discussing this topic, able to talk to those around you about this critical middle childhood phase. I believe every parent, caregiver, and educator who takes the time to understand these complex issues has the power to create a ripple of change in a child's life and the lives of those around them.

As you were reading, I imagine there were times when you stopped and remembered your own memories of feeling awkward during puberty—and maybe you were able to look back and laugh about them. I also know that there were likely times when you recalled how hard it was to figure out what was happening to your face, body, or friendships, perhaps without anyone to turn to. If this is true for you, I hope reading this book illuminated a way of beginning to reckon with the pain from your past. I can only hope that if this book brought back painful memories, such as hiding in your closet or crying in the school bathroom, you processed them so you can be even better able to respond instead of react, and that your child doesn't have to suffer as you did. Please don't hesitate to reach out to a trusted friend or even a therapist if you feel you need more support.

There is a saying in my field that "you can only take your child as far as you've gone yourself." My genuine wish for you is that you have learned enough, remembered a lot, and are now better positioned to recognize when your son is being picked on at school or your daughter wants a bra, or your child is suddenly showing signs of mental health issues. My hope is that you won't shy away from the tough talks with your child because you are emerging as a confident parent who understands why these changes occur and who has faith in your ability to handle them. I hope you are secure in the knowledge that the more confident you are, the more space your child will have to ask questions, share ideas, and simply wonder without pressure.

Childhood and adolescence are ongoing processes, and growth is lifelong for us all. As your child continues to develop, so too, will you. Although this book may end here, the journey continues, with each stage presenting new opportunities... though none quite like this one. The middle childhood years are truly the golden age of opportunity and I thank you for investing in them by reading this book and tuning in to your child's many needs. Ages six to twelve have long been known as the "forgotten years," but as you now know, they should be called the "crucial years" instead. Always remember, the work starts at home. The foundation gets laid by you; may you parent from a place of love—and not fear.

Acknowledgments

I walk in gratitude every day, and it brings me great joy to express my heartfelt appreciation to everyone who played a part in bringing my idea to life, once again.

First, to my incredible agent, Jen Marshall. This book would not have been born without you. Thank you for taking me on, for thoughtfully flushing out many ideas, and ultimately for having the belief in my work around puberty to guide me to write about it. You are brilliant, witty, sharp, and encouraging, and I am now glad to call you my friend.

My cowriter, Eve Claxton, you came in, immediately connected with me and the project, and changed the course and direction of the manuscript in ways that I am so grateful for. You eased any stress or doubts, you are calm and cool under pressure, and you know way too much about me! I am so happy that our paths were joined to put together a book that we can be proud of; thank you for your tireless work to make it just right. I look forward to many more years of sharing stories with one another.

My editors at Harvest, first Stephanie Fletcher: thank you for acquiring this book and believing in it. I hope that as your child approaches middle childhood you will find great joy in reading this book knowing that you played an important role in assuring that it was available to parents everywhere just when they need it. And to the great Sarah Pelz, I believe in synchronicity, I am sure you were meant to come back from your leave and have waiting on your desk a proposal from me about many of the things that you were about to go through! Your insights as a mom of kids in middle childhood, our long conversations about all things parenting, as well as your generous, tender, and kind heart allowed me the opportunity to create something special. Thank you for all your support and encouragement; working with you on this project has been a great blessing and privilege.

My sincere gratitude to Beth Chang, whose collaborative editorial skills were invaluable in helping to create the earliest versions of this book.

Eve Rodsky, just when I needed you, there you were at the start of the new year with a listening ear and an introduction to Jen. Thank you for that connection and knowing that we would be a great fit together. And most importantly, thank you for being authentically you—a gatherer of great minds, a fierce supporter of women, and an intentional community builder. I am forever grateful to be in your orbit.

My first editor, Carrie Thornton, your support over the past seven years has been invaluable. You have been a quiet angel, looking out for me and helping this second book become a reality. I see you. I thank you. I will always be grateful that you were my first editor. I hope this one makes you proud.

My first cowriter, Emily Klein, even though you didn't write this one you were with me every step of the way. Whether we are writing, talking, or learning from one another, I knew when I met you that we had a special connection. Thanks for being there when I needed direction, a listening ear, or a second reader, and for always making me feel seen and heard.

Kim Durand, without you, there would be no Start with the Talk, and my one-on-one conversations with kids would never have reached far and wide. Thank you for partnering with me to create something that has enriched the lives of countless girls and was the inspiration for this book.

Ashley Rodgers, thank you for sharing your expertise in the chapter on body image. Your comments and questions made the chapter and my message all the better, and for that I am grateful. My interns, Julia Lingelbach and Libby Schwalbach, it has been a pleasure to read your thoughtful edits and to listen to your fresh ideas. You are both intelligent young women with bright futures ahead of you in counseling and in writing.

Speaking of young women, to each and every girl who has taken this class a time or two, thank you for sharing your ideas and asking your important questions and for your vulnerability as you went from girl to young woman; this book would not exist without you. And I want to give special recognition to two schools in particular, Aspen Academy and Graland Country Day School, who have championed offering this course to their students, thank you for the support over the years. The champions behind this include my beautiful friends and leaders Shannon Bell, Erin Chain, and Kristina Scala—you are each incredible supporters of kids and mental health.

We all know it takes a village, so to the villagers who make up the behind-the-scenes team at Harvest, including Sharyn Rosenblum, Liz Psaltis, Emma

Effinger, and Deb Brody, thank you all for what you contributed both known and unknown to me. And to Ploy Siripant, who has now designed my second cover, thank you for another brilliant cover!

The team at Aevitas who supports Jen and therefore also supports me, including Erin Files, Vanessa Kerr, Kate Mack, Sam Babiak, Mags Chmielarczyk, and Lily Stephens, thank you for all you do for authors like me.

For my friends who ask me how the book is coming along, or if I included certain topics that you send me as links, or who lovingly tell me to hurry up because you need to read it—my heart is full. I am most grateful to my besties who support me and encourage me around book writing and ideas, including Allison Emig, Laura Whelan, Kirsten Gershon, Amy Reese, Jeannine Bernardi, and my cousin Aren Gonzalez—thank you, you have each stepped in at some point throughout the process when I needed it and I love you all for it.

To my mom, who normalized and celebrated puberty when I was a girl—thank you. To my aunt Ana, who was there for many milestones of my middle childhood—thanks for making it all feel okay. To my brother, Tommy, who was born when my middle childhood was ending, I adored you and hope you are smiling down from Heaven.

My husband, Steve—I am eternally grateful for your unconditional support, thank you for being my greatest cheerleader and always believing in me, I love you. And to my kids—I hope you will hold loving and fond memories from your crucial years; I gave it my all.

Notes

Introduction: Why Are These the Crucial Years?

1. Carol M. Worthman, Mark Tomlinson, and Mary Jane Rotheram-Borus, "When Can Parents Most Influence Their Child's Development? Expert Knowledge and Perceived Local Realities," *Social Science & Medicine* 154 (April 2016): 62–69, https://pubmed.ncbi.nlm.nih.gov/26945544.
2. Angela J. Beck et al., "Estimating the Distribution of the U.S. Psychiatric Subspecialist Workforce," University of Michigan School of Public Health Behavioral Health Workforce Research Center (2018), https://behavioralhealthworkforce.org/wp-content/uploads/2019/02/Y3-FA2-P2-Psych-Sub_Full-Report-FINAL2.19.2019.pdf.
3. Stacy Weiner, "A Growing Psychiatrist Shortage and an Enormous Demand for Mental Health Services," Association of American Medical Colleges, August 9, 2022, https://www.aamc.org/news/growing-psychiatrist-shortage-enormous-demand-mental-health-services.
4. Mohsen Saidinejad and Lois K. Lee, "Need to Improve Care of Children with Mental, Behavioral Health Emergencies Prompts New Joint Guidance," American Academy of Pediatrics (2023), https://publications.aap.org/aapnews/news/25397/Need-to-improve-care-of-children-with-mental.

Chapter 1: Middle Childhood and the Role of Parents

1. V. Kandice Mah and E. Lee Ford-Jones, "Spotlight on Middle Childhood: Rejuvenating the 'Forgotten Years,'" *Paediatrics & Child Health* 17, no. 2 (2012): 81–83, https://doi.org/10.1093/pch/17.2.81.
2. Rachel Maunder and Claire P. Monks, "Friendships in Middle Childhood: Links to Peer and School Identification, and General Self-Worth," British Psychological Society (2018), https://bpspsychub.onlinelibrary.wiley.com/doi/10.1111/bjdp.12268.
3. Sarah E. Lantz, "Freud's Developmental Theory," StatPearls Publishing, December 5, 2022. https://www.ncbi.nlm.nih.gov/books/NBK557526/.
4. Robin McKie, "Onset of Puberty in Girls Has Fallen by Five Years Since 1920," *The Guardian*, October 21, 2012, https://www.theguardian.com/society/2012/oct/21/puberty-adolescence-childhood-onset.
5. Rachel Maunder and Claire P. Monks, "Friendships in Middle Childhood: Links to Peer and School Identification, and General Self-Worth," *British Journal of Developmental Psychology* 37, no. 2 (2019): 211–29, https://doi.org/10.1111/bjdp.12268.

Chapter 2: The New Rules of Puberty

1. Elissa J. Hamlat et al., "Effects of Early Life Adversity on Pubertal Timing and Tempo in Black and White Girls: The National Growth and Health Study," *Psychosomatic Medicine*, April 1, 2023, https://pmc.ncbi.nlm.nih.gov/articles/PMC8976748/.
2. Ashraf Soliman, Vincenzo De Sanctis, Rania Elalaily, and Said Bedair, "Advances in Pubertal Growth and Factors Influencing It: Can We Increase Pubertal Growth?," *Indian Journal*

      of *Endocrinology and Metabolism* 18, Suppl 1 (2014): S53–S62, https://www.ncbi.nlm.nih.gov/pmc/articles/PMC4266869/.
3. Shauna Beni-Haynes, "14 Best Perfumes for Teens 2024," *Teen Vogue*, July 6, 2023, https://www.teenvogue.com/gallery/best-perfume-for-teens.
4. Mac Schwerin, "The Pungent Legacy of Axe Body Spray," *Vox*, February 12, 2020, https://www.vox.com/the-highlight/2020/2/12/21122543/axe-body-spray-teenage-boys-ads.
5. CS Mott Children's Hospital, "Masturbation and Young Children," Michigan Medicine, November 2020, https://www.mottchildren.org/posts/your-child/masturbation-and-young-children.
6. Bridget Sweet, "Voice Change and Singing Experiences of Adolescent Females," *Journal of Research in Music Education* 66, no. 2 (2018): 133–49, https://www.jstor.org/stable/48589035?seq=4.
7. Jane Mendle et al., "Family Structure and Age at Menarche: A Children-of-Twins Approach," *Developmental Psychology* 42, no. 3 (2006): 533–42, https://www.ncbi.nlm.nih.gov/pmc/articles/PMC2964498/.

Chapter 3: The Unexpected Ups and Downs of Middle Childhood: What Parents Can Do to Help

1. Keith Hamm, "Study Finds Parents' Phone Use in Front of Their Kids Can Harm Emotional Intelligence," *The Current*, March 10, 2023, https://news.ucsb.edu/2023/020867/screen-time-concerns.

Chapter 4: The Unexpected Emotional Ups and Downs of Middle Childhood: What Kids Can Do

1. Arianna Prothero, "Status Check: The Top Challenges to Social-Emotional Learning and How to Address Them," *Education Week*, 2023, https://www.edweek.org/teaching-learning/status-check-the-top-challenges-to-social-emotional-learning-and-how-to-address-them/2023/03.
2. Anne Trafton, "Practicing Mindfulness with an App May Improve Children's Mental Health," *MIT News*, 2023, https://news.mit.edu/2023/practicing-mindfulness-may-improve-childrens-mental-health-1011.
3. Harvard Health Publishing, "Yoga for Better Mental Health," 2024, https://www.health.harvard.edu/staying-healthy/yoga-for-better-mental-health.

Chapter 6: Understanding Sexual and Gender Identity Development

1. Kandace Redd, "Words Matter: A Guide to LGBTQIA+ Terminology," abc10.com, 2021, https://www.abc10.com/article/news/community/race-and-culture/a-guide-to-lgbtqia-terminology/103-5bf813a9-16e7-4a02-a591-c7de40dc7335.
2. Ibid.
3. Emily Mendelson, "The State of Sex Education in the USA in 2023," *Sex and Psychology*, March 22, 2023, https://www.sexandpsychology.com/blog/2023/3/22/the-state-of-sex-education-in-the-usa-in-2023/; Planned Parenthood, "State of Sex Education in USA | Health Education in Schools," n.d., https://www.plannedparenthood.org/learn/for-educators/whats-state-sex-education-us#:~:text=Currently%2C%2039%20states%20and%20the.
4. Katharine E. Kabotyanski and Leah H. Somerville. "Puberty: Your Brain on Hormones," *Frontiers for Young Minds*, February 2, 2021, https://kids.frontiersin.org/articles/10.3389/frym.2020.554380.
5. Sara Reardon, "Massive Study Finds No Single Genetic Cause of Same-Sex Sexual Behavior," *Scientific American*, August 29, 2019, https://www.scientificamerican.com/article/massive-study-finds-no-single-genetic-cause-of-same-sex-sexual-behavior/.

6. Pew Research Center, "Chapter 3: The Coming Out Experience," Social & Demographic Trends Project, June 13, 2013, https://www.pewresearch.org/social-trends/2013/06/13/chapter-3-the-coming-out-experience/.
7. Cambridge Dictionary, "Allyship," @CambridgeWords, July 5, 2023, https://dictionary.cambridge.org/us/dictionary/english/allyship.
8. American Academy of Pediatrics, "Mental Health in LGBTQ+ Youth: Pediatric Mental Health Minute Series," n.d., https://www.aap.org/en/patient-care/mental-health-minute/mental-health-in-lgbtq-youth/.
9. The Trevor Project, "Facts About LGBTQ Youth Suicide," 2024, https://www.thetrevorproject.org/resources/article/facts-about-lgbtq-youth-suicide/.
10. The Trevor Project, "2022 National Survey on LGBTQ Youth Mental Health," 2022, https://www.thetrevorproject.org/survey-2022/.
11. Chris Melore, "No Thanks: 1 in 5 Parents Say They'll Never Have 'the Talk' with Their Kids!," Study Finds, June 18, 2022, https://studyfinds.org/parents-birds-and-the-bees-kids/.
12. Supreet Mann, "Teens Are Watching Pornography, and It's Time to Talk About It," Common Sense Media, www.commonsensemedia.org, January 10, 2023, https://www.commonsensemedia.org/kids-action/articles/teens-are-watching-pornography-and-its-time-to-talk-about-it.
13. Michael Robb and Supreet Mann, "Teens and Pornography," Common Sense Media, 2022, https://www.commonsensemedia.org/sites/default/files/research/report/2022-teens-and-pornography-final-web.pdf.
14. USAFacts Team, "What Percentage of the US Population Is Transgender?," August 3, 2023, https://usafacts.org/articles/what-percentage-of-the-us-population-is-transgender/.
15. Cedars-Sinai, "Most Gender Dysphoria Established by Age 7," June 16, 2020, https://www.cedars-sinai.org/newsroom/most-gender-dysphoria-established-by-age-7-study-finds/.

Chapter 7: Body Image and Relationship with Food

1. Seeta Pai and Kelly Schryver, "Children, Teens, Media, and Body Image: A Common Sense Media Research Brief," Common Sense Media, 2015, https://www.commonsensemedia.org/sites/default/files/research/report/csm-body-image-report-012615-interactive.pdf.
2. Family Doctor editorial staff, "Body Image (Children and Teens)—Positive Body Image," familydoctor.org, April 23, 2019, https://familydoctor.org/building-your-childs-body-image-and-self-esteem/.
3. H. Klein and K. S. Shiffman, "Thin Is 'In' and Stout Is 'Out': What Animated Cartoons Tell Viewers About Body Weight," *Eating and Weight Disorders* 10, no. 2 (June 1, 2005): 107–16, https://doi.org/10.1007/BF03327532.
4. Kelly L. Klump, "Puberty as a Critical Risk Period for Eating Disorders: A Review of Human and Animal Studies," *Hormones and Behavior* 64, no. 2 (2013): 399–410, https://doi.org/10.1016/j.yhbeh.2013.02.019.
5. Mia Primeau, "Body Image: A Better Perspective," Stanford BeWell, June 18, 2020, https://bewell.stanford.edu/body-image-a-better-perspective/#:~:text=Your%20body%20image%20is%20defined%20by%20your%20personal.
6. Dario Cvencek, Anthony G. Greenwald, and Andrew N. Meltzoff, "Implicit Measures for Preschool Children Confirm Self-Esteem's Role in Maintaining a Balanced Identity," *Journal of Experimental Social Psychology* 62 (January 2016): 50–57, https://doi.org/10.1016/j.jesp.2015.09.015.
7. Ulrich Orth, Ruth Yasmin Erol, and Eva C. Luciano (2018). "Development of Self-Esteem from Age 4 to 94 Years: A Meta-Analysis of Longitudinal Studies." Psychological Bulletin, 144, no. 10: 1045–1080. https://doi.org/10.1037/bul0000161.
8. National Association of Anorexia Nervosa and Associated Disorders, "Body Shaming: What It Is and How to Overcome It," April 5, 2019, https://anad.org/get-informed/body-image/body-image-articles/body-shaming/#:~:text=Body%20shaming%20is%20known%20as.

9. Substance Abuse and Mental Health Services Administration, "Table 23, DSM-IV to DSM-5 Body Dysmorphic Disorder Comparison," National Institutes of Health, June 2016, https://www.ncbi.nlm.nih.gov/books/NBK519712/table/ch3.t19/.
10. Anxiety & Depression Association of America, "Body Dysmorphic Disorder (BDD)," 2021, https://adaa.org/understanding-anxiety/body-dysmorphic-disorder; Mental Health America, "Body Dysmorphic Disorder (BDD) and Youth," n.d., https://www.mhanational.org/body-dysmorphic-disorder-bdd-and-youth.
11. Avneet Kaur, Ashishjot Kaur, and Gaurav Singla, "Rising Dysmorphia Among Adolescents: A Cause for Concern," *Journal of Family Medicine and Primary Care* 9, no. 2 (February 28, 2020): 567–70, https://doi.org/10.4103/jfmpc.jfmpc_738_19.
12. Amita Jassi and Georgina Krebs, "Body Dysmorphic Disorder: Reflections on the Last 25 Years," *Clinical Child Psychology and Psychiatry* 26, no. 1 (January 2021): 3–7, https://doi.org/10.1177/1359104520984818.
13. Ibid.
14. Beth A Abramovitz and Leann L Birch, "Five-Year-Old Girls' Ideas About Dieting Are Predicted by Their Mothers' Dieting," *Journal of the American Dietetic Association* 100, no. 10 (October 2000): 1157–63, https://doi.org/10.1016/s0002-8223(00)00339-4; Charlotte M. Handford, Ronald M. Rapee, and Jasmine Fardouly, "The Influence of Maternal Modeling on Body Image Concerns and Eating Disturbances in Preadolescent Girls," *Behaviour Research and Therapy* 100 (January 2018): 17–23, https://doi.org/10.1016/j.brat.2017.11.001.
15. Stuart B. Murray, Aaron J. Blashill, and Jerel P. Calzo, "Prevalence of Disordered Eating and Associations with Sex, Pubertal Maturation, and Weight in Children in the US," *JAMA Pediatrics*, August 1, 2022, https://doi.org/10.1001/jamapediatrics.2022.2490.
16. National Institute of Mental Health, "Eating Disorders," 2024, https://www.nimh.nih.gov/health/topics/eating-disorders.
17. David B. Sarwer, Carlos M. Grilo, and Anne E. Kazak, eds., *Obesity: Psychosocial and Behavioral Aspects of a Modern Epidemic* 75, no. 2 (2020), https://www.apa.org/pubs/journals/special/amp-obesity-psychosocial-behavioral-aspects-pdf.
18. David B. Sarwer and Heather M. Polonsky, "The Psychosocial Burden of Obesity," *Endocrinology and Metabolism Clinics of North America* 45, no. 3 (July 19, 2018): 677–88, https://doi.org/10.1016/j.ecl.2016.04.016.
19. Obesity Medicine Association. "Why Is Obesity a Disease?," December 30, 2023, https://obesitymedicine.org/blog/why-is-obesity-a-disease/.
20. Zhe Fang et al., "Association of Ultra-Processed Food Consumption with All Cause and Cause Specific Mortality: Population Based Cohort Study," *BMJ* 385 (May 8, 2024): e078476, https://doi.org/10.1136/bmj-2023-078476.
21. Eric M. Hecht et al., "Cross-Sectional Examination of Ultra-Processed Food Consumption and Adverse Mental Health Symptoms," *Public Health Nutrition* 25, no. 11 (July 28, 2022): 1–10, https://doi.org/10.1017/s1368980022001586.
22. Beth A. Abramovitz and Leann L. Birch, "Five-Year-Old Girls' Ideas About Dieting Are Predicted by Their Mothers' Dieting," *Journal of the American Dietetic Association* 100, no. 10 (October 2000): 1157–63, https://doi.org/10.1016/s0002-8223(00)00339-4.
23. Lu Wang et al., "Trends in Consumption of Ultraprocessed Foods Among US Youths Aged 2–19 Years, 1999–2018," *JAMA* 326, no. 6 (August 10, 2021): 519. https://doi.org/10.1001/jama.2021.10238.
24. Juliana Bunim, "Cutting Sugar from Kids' Diets Improves Health in Just Days," University of California, October 27, 2015, https://www.universityofcalifornia.edu/news/cutting-sugar-kids-diets-improves-health-just-days#:~:text=After%20just%20nine%20days%20on.
25. Rosanna Turner, "What Is Intuitive Eating? A Nutritionist Explains," Cedars-Sinai, March 8, 2021, https://www.cedars-sinai.org/blog/what-is-intuitive-eating.html; "What Is Intuitive Eating? 10 Principles to Follow," Cleveland Clinic, June 8, 2022, https://health.clevelandclinic.org/what-is-intuitive-eating.

26. Ivonne P. M. Derks et al., "Early Childhood Appetitive Traits and Eating Disorder Symptoms in Adolescence: A 10-Year Longitudinal Follow-Up Study in the Netherlands and the UK," *The Lancet*, February 24, 2024, https://www.thelancet.com/journals/lanchi/article/PIIS2352-4642(23)00342-5/fulltext.
27. Ibid.

Chapter 8: Preteens and Success: Shaping Healthier Digital Habits

1. Common Sense Media, "Two Years into the Pandemic, Media Use Has Increased 17% Among Tweens and Teens," March 23, 2022, https://www.commonsensemedia.org/press-releases/two-years-into-the-pandemic-media-use-has-increased-17-among-tweens-and-teens.
2. Caraline McDonnell, "A Tech-Based World: The Risks and Benefits of Social Media and Screentime," Baker Center for Children and Families, November 7, 2023, https://www.bakercenter.org/screentime-1#:~:text=As%20of%202022%2C%20up%20to.
3. Precise, "Kids and the Screen: Changing the Channel," Giraffe Insights, 2021, https://content.precise.tv/hubfs/pdf/PreciseTV_Kids_and_the_Screen_USA.pdf.
4. Kelsey Ables, "New York City Designates Social Media a Public Health Hazard," *Washington Post*, January 25, 2024, https://www.washingtonpost.com/technology/2024/01/25/nyc-social-media-health-hazard-toxin/.
5. Emily Dreyfuss, "Opinion: Our Kids Are Living in a Different Digital World." *New York Times*, January 12, 2024, https://www.nytimes.com/2024/01/12/opinion/children-nicotine-zyn-social-media.html.
6. Jenny S. Radesky et al., "Constant Companion: A Week in the Life of a Young Person's Smartphone Use," Common Sense Media, September 26, 2023, https://www.commonsensemedia.org/research/constant-companion-a-week-in-the-life-of-a-young-persons-smartphone-use.
7. Trevor Haynes, "Dopamine, Smartphones & You: A Battle for Your Time," Science in the News, Harvard University, May 1, 2018, https://sitn.hms.harvard.edu/flash/2018/dopamine-smartphones-battle-time/; Needa Qureshi, "Dopamine and Social Media: The Science Behind Scrolling for Hours," brain-feed.com, June 14, 2023, https://brain-feed.com/blogs/the-science/dopamine-and-social-media-the-science-behind-scrolling-for-hours.
8. Hezu Liu et al., "Screen Time and Childhood Attention Deficit Hyperactivity Disorder: A Meta-Analysis," *Reviews on Environmental Health* 39, no 4. (May 11, 2023), https://doi.org/10.1515/reveh-2022-0262.
9. Tate Ryan-Mosley, "A High School's Deepfake Porn Scandal Is Pushing US Lawmakers into Action," *MIT Technology Review*, December 1, 2023, https://www.technologyreview.com/2023/12/01/1084164/deepfake-porn-scandal-pushing-us-lawmakers/.
10. Jessica A. Kent, "Need a Break from Social Media? Here's Why You Should—and How to Do It," Harvard Summer School, May 8, 2023. https://summer.harvard.edu/blog/need-a-break-from-social-media-heres-why-you-should-and-how-to-do-it/.
11. Martin Korte, "The Impact of the Digital Revolution on Human Brain and Behavior: Where Do We Stand?," *Dialogues in Clinical Neuroscience* 22, no. 2 (June 1, 2020): 101–11, https://doi.org/10.31887/DCNS.2020.22.2/mkorte.
12. FTC Bureau of Consumer Protection, "FTC Video Game Loot Box Workshop," August 2020, https://www.ftc.gov/system/files/documents/reports/staff-perspective-paper-loot-box-workshop/loot_box_workshop_staff_perspective.pdf.
13. Heather Stewart, "'Our Kids Are Suffering': Calls for Ban on Social Media to Protect Under-16s," *The Guardian*, February 11, 2024, https://www.theguardian.com/media/2024/feb/11/our-kids-are-suffering-calls-for-ban-on-social-media-to-protect-under-16s.
14. College of Arts and Sciences, "Study Shows Habitual Checking of Social Media May Impact Young Adolescents' Brain Development," University of North Carolina at Chapel Hill, January 3, 2023,

https://www.unc.edu/posts/2023/01/03/study-shows-habitual-checking-of-social-media-may-impact-young-adolescents-brain-development/.
15. Martin Korte, "The Impact of the Digital Revolution on Human Brain and Behavior: Where Do We Stand?," *Dialogues in Clinical Neuroscience* 22, no. 2 (June 1, 2020): 101–11, https://doi.org/10.31887/DCNS.2020.22.2/mkorte.
16. "Toxic Beauty Standards on Social Media: The Stats," www.dove.com, November 2, 2023, https://www.dove.com/us/en/stories/campaigns/social-media-and-body-image.html#:~:text=Toxic%20beauty%20advice%20normalizes%20unrealistic.
17. Instagram, "Teen Safety Tips for Parents," n.d., https://about.instagram.com/community/parents.

Chapter 9: Substances

1. Majed M. Ramadan, Jim E. Banta, Khaled Bahjri, and Susanne B. Montgomery, "Frequency of Cannabis Use and Alcohol-Associated Adverse Effects in a Representative Sample of U.S. Adolescents and Youth (2002–2014) a Cross-Sectional Study," *Journal of Cannabis Research* 2, no. 1 (October 20, 2020), https://doi.org/10.1186/s42238-020-00043-z.
2. Alexis Wnuck, "Is Cannabis Today Really Much More Potent than 50 Years Ago?," *New Scientist*, October 11, 2023, https://www.newscientist.com/article/2396976-is-cannabis-today-really-much-more-potent-than-50-years-ago/.
3. Sara Ali, Mina Sardashti, and Shawn Sidhu, "Marijuana Use in Teens," University of New Mexico's Health Sciences Center Newsroom, June 21, 2019, https://hsc.unm.edu/news/news/marijuana-use-in-teens.html.
4. Joanna Jacobus and Susan F. Tapert, "Effects of Cannabis on the Adolescent Brain," *Current Pharmaceutical Design* 20, no. 13 (2014): 2186–93, https://doi.org/10.2174/13816128113199990426.
5. Julie Wernau, "More Teens Who Use Marijuana Are Suffering from Psychosis," *Wall Street Journal*, January 11, 2024, https://www.wsj.com/us-news/marijuana-depression-psychosis-8694900d1.
6. Mariliis Tael-Oeren, "Parents' Lenient Attitudes Towards Drinking Linked to Greater Alcohol Use Among Childre," University of Cambridge, June 12, 2019, https://www.cam.ac.uk/research/news/parents-lenient-attitudes-towards-drinking-linked-to-greater-alcohol-use-among-children.
7. National Institute on Alcohol Abuse and Alcoholism, "Underage Drinking," February 2024, https://www.niaaa.nih.gov/publications/brochures-and-fact-sheets/underage-drinking.
8. Bridget F. Grant and Deborah A. Dawson, "Age of Onset of Drug Use and Its Association with DSM-IV Drug Abuse and Dependence: Results from the National Longitudinal Alcohol Epidemiologic Survey," *Journal of Substance Abuse* 10, no. 2 (January 1998): 163–73, https://doi.org/10.1016/s0899-3289(99)80131-x.
9. Substance Abuse and Mental Health Services, "Why You Should Talk with Your Child About Alcohol and Other Drugs," www.samhsa.gov, September 27, 2022, https://www.samhsa.gov/talk-they-hear-you/parent-resources/why-you-should-talk-your-child.
10. National Institute on Drug Abuse, "Monitoring the Future," December 15, 2021, https://nida.nih.gov/research-topics/trends-statistics/monitoring-future.
11. Allison L. Groom, "The Influence of Friends on Teen Vaping: A Mixed-Methods Approach," *International Journal of Environmental Research and Public Health* 18, no. 13 (June 24, 2021): 6784, https://doi.org/10.3390/ijerph18136784.
12. Hannah Messinger, "Learning and the Teen Brain: Driving, SATs, and Addiction," Penn Medicine, August 30, 2018, https://www.pennmedicine.org/news/news-blog/2018/august/learning-and-the-teen-brain-driving-sats-and-addiction.

Index

abdominal cramps and menstruation, 81–82
abortion, 11, 48, 176, 177
absenteeism. *See* school absenteeism
abstinence, 275, 278
academic pressures. *See* school pressure
acceptance and commitment therapy (ACT), 129–30
acne, 78–80
   BDD and, 206, 207
   menstruation and, 81
   script for talking about, 78–80
ACOAs (adult children of alcoholics), 278
active listening, 107–8
active parenting, stages of, 33–34
active shooter drills, 3, 157–58
Adam's apples, 73
Adams, Jerome, 282
addiction, 284–85. *See also* substance abuse
   screens, 235, 238, 240–42, 256–61
ADHD (attention deficit hyperactivity disorder), 13, 242–43
   screen time and, 242–43
   substance abuse and, 273
adolescence, 2, 4–5, 34. *See also* middle childhood
   age of, 2, 8, 22, 49
   changes in, 34–35
   friendships in, 21
   gender identity development, 180
   global youth mental health crisis, 9–13
adrenal glands, 52–53
adrenaline, 99, 158
adrenarche, 53
adultification, 61–62
affirmations, 101, 134
ages and stages in middle childhood, 25–33
   six, 25–27, 180
   seven, 27–28, 180
   eight, 28–29, 180
   nine, 29–30, 180

ten, 30–3, 180
eleven and twelve, 32–33, 180
aggression
   authoritarian parenting style and, 40
   developmental stages, 26
   gender differences and social constructs, 88, 181
   hyper-arousal and, 94
   physical bullying, 148, 151
   video games and, 256
alcohol (alcohol use disorder), 278–81
   Leah and Joel's story, 278–79
   talking to child about, 280–81
algorithms, social media, 261–62, 272
alternative solutions, 124–25
Amanat, Soroosh, 160–61
American Academy of Pediatrics (AAP), 10–13, 49, 159, 160, 170, 219, 225, 256
American Girl Wellbeing, 58
American Psychological Association (APA), 12, 140, 141, 170
amygdala, 132, 135, 235
androgens, 53, 78
anger
   identifying, 119, 122
   identifying triggers, 123
   parents and co-regulation, 96–98
   parents and mindfulness, 98–100
   parents and "tear and repair," 102–3
   Ryan's meltdowns, 88, 89, 90, 116–18
   "Stop and Think" for, 130, 131
   the Volcano, 126–27, 127
   window of tolerance and, 94
Angier, Natalie, 16
anorexia nervosa, 212, 215, 216
anticipatory anxiety, 55
antiperspirants, 52, 67–68
anxiety
   authoritarian parenting style and, 40
   avoidance and, 134, 140, 215
   body image and, 191–92, 206, 207, 213, 215

anxiety (*continued*)
  Cici's story, 139–43
  earlier puberty in girls and, 48
  Emilia's story, 272
  emotional regulation, 92, 94, 113, 116, 134
  global youth mental health crisis and, 9–13
  Hannah, Chris and Brandon's story, 19–20, 21, 35, 37–38, 42–43, 44
  hyper-arousal and, 94
  Leila's story, 191–92
  LGBTQ+ children and, 173
  mindfulness for, 134
  obesity and, 219
  physical activity and sports for, 160–61, 162
  rising incidence of, 10, 11
  school. *See* school anxiety
  social media and screens, 234, 235, 237, 272
  substance abuse and, 273, 284–85
  UPFs and, 223
Anxiety Center, 141
apologies, 57, 103, 152
appearance, 201–2. *See also* body image
  beauty culture, 265–66
  commenting on children's bodies, 197–98
  girls and gender differences, 32, 194–95
  promoting health versus, 225
  self-esteem connection, 199–201, 202
apps, 262–63
  AI and, 253
  educational, 231
  meditation, 135
  mental health, 193
  parental controls, 237, 245, 246, 250, 252, 257, 269
  privacy concerns, 250, 263
  weight-loss, 226
areola, 73–74
Are You There God? It's Me, Margaret (movie), 74
artificial intelligence (AI), 36, 253–54
asynchronous development, 37
attention deficit hyperactivity disorder. *See* ADHD
"attention economy," 262–63
attention regulation, 132–33, 134
attention spans, 20, 92
  age six, 27
  age seven, 28
  age eight, 29
  age nine, 30
  age ten, 32
  ages eleven and twelve, 33
  screen time and, 102, 242–43

"attitude of gratitude," 101
attunement, 104–7
authoritarian parenting style, 39–40, 42
authoritative parenting style, 38–39, 42
autonomy, 35, 144–45, 163, 175, 188
avoidance, 134, 215
  anxiety and, 140, 152–58, 215
avoidant restrictive food intake disorder (ARFID), 216–17

baby teeth and Tooth Fairy, 24–25
"bad" foods, 226, 230
Bandura, Albert, 96
Barbie, 191, 210
bathing suits, 192, 203
Baumrind, Diana, 38
beauty culture, 210, 265–66
bedtime, 88, 121, 156
  screen time and, 239–40, 246, 248
Be Internet Awesome, 249
belly breathing, 99–100, 133
Benjamin, Harry, 187
binge-eating disorder, 215
biological sex, 180–81, 185, 186
bisexual, 165, 170, 173
Black children, 13, 48, 60–62, 219
blaming, 112
bleaching hair, 69
blended households, and menstruation talk, 82
bloating, 81–82
blue light glasses, 240
body awareness, 135–37
body development, 45–84
  acne, 78–80
  ages, 47–50, 52, 53
  answering child's questions, 65–66
  Ava's story, 45–46, 49
  body odor, 67–69
  boys and breasts, 75
  boy's reproductive system, 70–72
  coping strategies for helping child navigate, 83–84
  FAQs, 52–55
  first signs and symptoms, 53–55
  girls and menstruation, 80–83
  girls' breast development, 53–54, 59, 73–74
  girls' reproductive system, 59, 75, 76, 77–78
  hair, 69–70
  height and weight, 66–67
  paradigm shift, 51

Index

parental comfort talking about, 45–47, 50–51, 55–60. *See also* "Talk, The"
race and earlier puberty, 48, 60–62
sex scripts, 62–65
voice changes and Adam's apples, 73
body dysmorphic disorder (BDD), 191–92, 206–11
   age of symptom onset, 206
   Leila's story, 191–94, 195, 206
   red flags, 196, 202–3, 204, 207–8
body fat, 67, 74
body hair, 52, 69–70
body image, 191–230
   beauty culture, 265–66
   commenting on children's bodies, 197–98
   development of, 198
   issues facing, 201–8
   Leila's story, 191–94, 195, 206
   paradigm shift, 196–97
   parental support of positive sense of, 208–11
   primer on, 198–99
   relationship with food, 211–28
   self-esteem connection, 199–201, 202
   signs and red flags, 196, 202–3
   social media and, 194, 198–99
body language, 106, 108, 136, 152
body odor, 52–53, 67–69
   sample script, 68–69
"body scans," 136
body shaming, 203–5, 230
body sprays, 52, 67
"boner," 71
books, recommended, 58, 74
boredom, 39, 40, 43, 235
boundary setting
   body changes and, 47
   Cici and school work, 142
   parenting and, 33, 34, 37–39, 87, 138, 175
box breathing, 133
boys
   body image, 195, 229
   brain changes, 54–55
   breasts and, 75
   puberty in, 2, 49–50, 52–53, 54–55, 59–60, 64–65
   puberty talk with, 59–60
   reproductive system, 70–72
   sex talk with, 64–65
   social constructs, 181–83
brain (brain development)
   emotions and, 88, 89, 91–93, 99
   mindfulness and, 134, 135

puberty and, 49, 52, 54–55
screen time and, 235–36, 243, 260–61
brain plasticity, 91–92, 99
brain training, 124–25
bras, 2, 45–46, 55, 74
Brazilian waxes, 69
breast buds, 2, 37, 45–46, 53–54, 60–62, 66, 73–74, 77
breast cancer and deodorants, 67–68
breast development, 50, 52–54, 73–74, 168
   Ava's story, 45–46, 49
   race and earlier puberty, 60–62
   "The Talk" about, 59, 66
breast nipples, 53, 73–74
breasts and boys, 75
breathing, 99–100, 132–33
bulimia nervosa, 212, 215, 216
bullying, 147–52, 155–56
   body shaming, 203–5
   consequences of, 149–50
   cyberbullying, 148, 236, 254–55
   elements of, 147–48
   incidence of, 149
   of LGBTQ+ children, 173–74
   preventing child from being the bully, 150–52
   social constructs for boys and, 182
   types of, 148–49
   use of term, 147–48
burnout, 141, 159, 163
   Cici's story, 139–43
business models, online, 262–63
busyness, 43, 113, 142

calming, 89, 97, 99, 156, 183
cancer, 48, 67–68, 219, 236, 284
car seats, 236
Cauldwell, David, 187
CBD (cannabidiol), 272, 276
cell phones. *See* apps; screen time; smartphones
Centers for Disease Control (CDC), 9, 10, 11, 47, 49, 50, 219, 275
cerebral cortex, 132, 134
cervix, 76, 77
challenging parenthood, 34
childhood obesity, 2, 61, 197, 218–22, 223
   Ella's story, 218–19, 220–22
   epidemic of, 48, 219
   terminology, 219–20
Child Protective Services (CPS), 153
child psychologists, shortage in, 12–13
Children's Hospital Association, 10

Index

circadian rhythms, 240
circumcision, 70–71
cisgender, 165, 166
Cleveland Clinic, 12, 68, 243
climate change, 3
clothing. *See* dress and clothing
Columbine High School shooting, 3, 157
Common Sense Media, 177, 240, 246, 249
Common Sense Media Digital Literacy and Citizenship, 249
competency, 26, 35–37
"conceptualizing challenging situations," 112
consent, 174–75, 177, 188
consistency, 42, 94–95, 114, 218
containment, 111–12
contraception, 175–76, 177
Controlled Substances Act, 277
"conversion therapy," 171
co-parenting, 90
co-regulation, 96–98, 117
cortisol, 21, 156, 160, 267
Couric, Katie, 274
COVID-19 pandemic, 3, 9–10, 11, 48, 154
crushes, 168–69
crying, 37, 87–88, 144
   identifying triggers, 123
   parents and emotional regulation, 96, 103, 108, 111
cyberbullying, 148, 236, 254–55

dancing, 28, 121, 135, 136, 262
decentering, 129–30
deepfakes, 253–54
demisexual, 165
deodorants, 52, 67–68
depression
   body image and, 194, 206, 207, 209, 213, 215, 218–19, 223
   earlier puberty in girls and, 48
   Ella's story, 218–19
   global youth mental health crisis and, 9–13
   LGBTQ+ children and, 13, 173
   obesity and, 218–19
   parenting styles and, 40
   perfectionism and parental pressure, 140–42
   physical activity and sports for, 160–61, 162
   rising incidence of, 10
   self-regulation, 92
   social media and screens, 234, 235, 237, 260, 261
   substance abuse and, 273, 276
   team sport participation for, 160–61
   UPFs and, 223
development
   of body. *See* body development
   sexual. *See* sexual development
   of sexual identities, 168–70
developmental stages, 8–9, 20–33
   by age, 25–33. *See also* ages and stages in middle childhood
   gender identities, 179–80
   psychological theories, 22–25, 34–35
diabetes, 219, 223
Diagnostic and Statistical Manual of Mental Health Disorders (DSM-5), 242
dialectical behavior therapy (DBT), 89
diaphragmatic breathing, 99–100, 133
diet. *See also* food
   processed and ultra-processed foods, 222–24, 230
   restrictive, 199, 202, 211, 212, 214–15, 216, 226
   sugar, 224–25
dieting, 195, 199, 211, 213, 225, 229
digital citizenship, 210, 248–50
digital detox, 267–68
digital footprint, 263–64
digital habits. *See* screen time
digital literacy, 249, 269
digital sundown, 240
dinner table. *See* mealtimes
discovery parenthood, 33
discrimination, 13, 173–74
disgust, 45, 81, 119, 122
disordered eating behavior (DEB), 211–16
   Keiran's story, 211–14
   Leila's story, 192–94, 195
   paradigm shift, 196–97
   red flags, 214–15
   risk factors, 213
   signs and red flags, 196, 212–13
divorced households, and menstruation talk, 80, 82
dopamine, 102, 240–42
dress and clothing, 209–10
   BDD and, 207, 209–10
   gender expression and, 165–66, 183–84
drinking. *See* alcohol

earlier puberty, 2, 14, 21, 48–51
   coping strategies for helping child navigate, 83–84

FAQs, 52–55
race and, 48, 60–62
eating. *See also* diet; food
  picky eaters, 216, 217–18
eating disorders, 198, 212–13, 228–29
  anorexia nervosa/bulimia, 212, 215, 216
  ARFID, 216–17
  BDD and, 192–93, 206, 212
  disordered eating vs., 212
  Leila's story, 193–94, 195
  perfectionism and parental pressure, 140–42
  risk factors, 215–16
  signs and red flags, 196, 212–13
eating habits, 214–15, 220, 221
e-cigarettes (vaping), 281–83
educational video games, 255–56
ejaculation, 71–72
Ekman, Paul, 119
embarrassment
  Ava's story, 45
  bullying and, 148, 254, 255
  digital footprint and, 254, 255, 263
  food and avoidance, 215
  identifying, 120, 122
  puberty and acne, 79
  puberty and body changes, 45, 47, 50, 51, 55
  puberty and body odor, 68
  puberty and sex, 57, 71–72, 80
  Ryan's story, 88
emojis, 119–20, 122
emotions and food, 209, 227–28
emotions, identifying, 119–22
  facial expressions, 119–20, 122
emotional check-ins, 121, 209
emotional dysregulation, 89–90, 108–9
  child's window of tolerance, 93–96
  identifying emotions, 119–20
  signs and red flags, 118
emotional eating, 214
emotional intelligence, 26, 92, 102, 145
emotional literacy tools, 120
emotional regulation, 87–138
  of child. *See* emotional regulation of child
  paradigm shifts, 91, 119
  parents and. *See* emotional regulation and parents
emotional regulation and parents, 88–89, 96–115
  active listening, 107–8
  attunement, 104–7
  "conceptualizing challenging situations," 112
  co-regulation and self-regulation, 96–98

intention setting, 100–101
love vs. fear, 113–14
mantras, 101
mindfulness techniques, 98–102
monotasking, 101–2
reactive vs. responsive parenting, 110–11
signs and red flags, 90
"tear and repair," 102–3
validation, 108–10
"Who holds the energy here?", 104
emotional regulation of child, 88–89, 116–38
  alternative solutions, 124–25
  body awareness, 135–37
  brain and, 88, 89, 91–93, 99
  containment, 111–12
  identifying emotions, 119–22
  identifying triggers and proactive planning, 123–25
  mindfulness techniques, 132–35
  Ryan, Jaime and Greg's story, 87–90, 92, 93–94, 108, 116–17, 120, 123, 129
  sense of control, 123, 131–32
  signs and red flags, 118
  Stop, Breathe, Think, Then Act, 130–31, 137
  thought replacements, 125–26
  tools for, 119–22
  visual metaphors, 126–30
  window of tolerance, 93–96, 95
emotional synchronicity, 105
empathy, 8, 35, 137–38, 150–52
  attunement and, 105
  building, 151–52
  bullying and, 150–52
  validation and, 109, 110
"empathy gap," 150–51
endorphins, 134, 160, 225
entrainment, 97–98
erections, 54, 71–72
Erikson, Erik, 23–24, 34–35
estrogen, 52, 223
euphemisms, 47, 57, 81
exercise. *See also* sports
  benefits of, 161, 225
  body dysmorphia and, 196, 202, 207
  body image and, 220, 225
exploration parenthood, 34
eyestrain, 240

Facebook, 241, 260
facial expressions, 119–20, 122
facial hair, 52, 69–70

fallopian tubes, 64, 75, 76, 77, 81
family game nights, 237
fast food, 193, 194
"fat," 192–96, 202, 219
"fat jokes," 204
fear (fear response), 113–14, 119
feminine hygiene products, 49, 55, 82
fentanyl, 275, 276
fight, flight, or freeze response, 94, 99, 132, 227
follicle-stimulating hormone, 52
FOMO (fear of missing out), 267
food
　body image and relationship with, 195, 196, 211–28
　childhood obesity. *See* childhood obesity
　eating disorders. *See* eating disorders
　feelings and, 209, 227–28
　as fuel, 227, 230
　Leila's story, 191–94, 195, 206
　mealtimes. *See* mealtimes
　parental communication about, 225–28
　picky eaters, 216, 217–18
　processed and ultra-processed foods, 48, 222–24, 230
　sugar, 224–25, 230
food judgment, 226–27
"food mood," 227
food responsiveness, 228
Ford-Jones, E. Lee, 20
four, seven, eight breathing technique, 133
free play. *See* play
Freud, Sigmund, 22–23
friendships, 2, 11, 20, 35, 89, 201
　age seven, 27
　age eight, 28
　age nine, 29
　age ten, 30–31
　ages eleven and twelve, 32
　Brandon's story, 21
frustration, 1, 29, 38, 89, 90, 94, 97, 98, 116, 119, 124, 137

Galinsky, Ellen, 33
gambling, online, 258–59
gamma-aminobutyric acid (GABA), 134
gay. *See* LGBTQ+
gay gene, 170–71
gay insults, 172–73
gender binary, 14, 165
gender differences
　in body image, 191, 194–95, 197
　in body odor, 67
　in confidence, 32
　in puberty, 2, 49–50, 52–55
　social constructs, 181–82
gender dysphoria, 186–87
gender expression, 183–84
gender identity, 3–4, 14, 164–66, 178–88
　author's story, 164–65
　paradigm shift, 167
　signs and red flags, 167
　social constructs, 180–83
　"stages" of development, 179–80
　use of term, 178–79
gender nonconformity, 165, 184–86
　Skye's story, 184–85
gender pronoun usage, 14
gender stereotypes, 181–82, 210
genetics
　body development and, 67, 70, 74, 79
　body size and obesity, 203, 220
　DEB and, 213
　food responsiveness and, 228
　sexual orientation, 170–71
genitals, 46–47, 54, 57, 63–64, 70–71
"Get Ready with Me" routines, 194–95
G.I. Joe, 210
girls
　body image, 191, 194–95, 197, 210, 229
　brain changes, 54–55
　breast development. *See* breast development
　menstruation. *See* menstruation
　puberty, 2, 49–50, 52–55, 59, 63–64
　puberty talk with, 57, 59
　reproductive system, 75, 76, 77–78
　sex talk with, 63–64
　social constructs, 182–83
global youth mental health crisis, 4, 9–13
goal setting, 36
gonadotropin, 52
"good" foods, 226, 230
Good Housekeeping, 144–45
Google, 45–46, 188
　Be Internet Awesome, 249
Google Kids Space, 251
Gottman, John, 104–5
gratitude, 101
Greene, Ross, 139
group chats, 231, 233, 239, 254, 268
growing pains, 10, 66–67
growth mindset, 199
guessing game, 120–21

Index

guilt, 29, 31, 38, 128, 213, 214, 226, 239, 241
gut health, 223
gynecomastia, 75

hair, 52, 69–70
Hamm, Jon, 270
Hancock, Jeff, 260
heart disease, 219, 284
heart rate, 99, 136, 241
height changes, 54, 66–67
highly gifted and talented (HGT), 141
hippocampus, 91, 134
Hirschfeld, Magnus, 187
Hispanic children, 60–62, 219
hydration, 225
hygiene
    body odor and, 67–69
    feminine products, 49, 55, 82
    skin problems and, 78
hyper-arousal, 94, 223
hypo-arousal, 94
hypothalamus, 52

Iceberg, the, 128–29
impaired judgment and marijuana, 276
influencer culture, 264–66
Inside Out (movie), 45, 116
Instagram, 233, 234, 241, 260, 265
insulin, 220, 223
insults, 118, 148, 172–73
intention setting, 56–57, 100–101
intrusive thoughts, 193
intuition, 137
iPhones. *See* screen time; smartphones

"jerking off," 71
jobs, 146
journaling, 28, 31, 121, 193
joy, 15, 24, 45, 113, 119
JUUL, 282

Kessler, David, 113
kindness, 141, 146, 150, 151, 163
Knost, L. R., 19
Kübler-Ross, Elisabeth, 113

labia, 53, 77
larynx (voice box), 73
latency stage, 22–23
leg hair, 52, 69–70
leptin, 220

LGBTQ+, 165, 170–74, 188. *See also* sexual identity
    mental health concerns, 13, 173–74, 185, 188
    teaching child to be an ally, 172–73
limbic system, 91, 235, 283
Linehan, Marsha, 89
"loot boxes," 258–59
love response, 113–14
luteinizing hormone, 52

Mah, V. Kandice, 20
"male effect," 82
mantras, 101, 134
marijuana, 273–77
    Emilia and Celeste's story, 271–73
    harms, 274–75
    how to talk to your child about, 276–77
    legalization of, 273–74, 276
masturbation, 71, 72
maternal stress, 220, 243
mealtimes
    body image and, 226
    emotional dysregulation and, 118
    food and avoidance, 215
    Keiran's story, 213–14
    picky eaters and, 218
    Ryan's story, 88
    screen time at, 237
media literacy, 210, 249, 269
medications, 13, 215, 272, 276
meditation, 101, 135
melatonin, 240
meltdowns, 36–37, 88, 89, 96, 116–18, 131. *See also* anger
menarche, 53
menstruation (period), 45, 46, 47, 49–50, 77–78, 80–83, 168
    Andie's story, 80
    Gabby's story, 80
    script for talking about, 81–83
mental health
    barriers to treatment, 11–13
    body image and, 193, 195, 206, 209, 213
    bullying and, 149, 254
    childhood obesity and, 219
    global youth crisis in, 4, 9–13
    of LGBTQ+ children, 13, 173–74, 185, 188
    low self-esteem and, 35, 172
    marijuana and, 277
    obesity and, 219
    parental role, 13–14, 41
    race and, 13, 61

mental health (*continued*)
   school pressures and, 140, 142, 143, 147, 154, 157, 158
   social media and screens, 234, 236, 259–60
   sport participation for, 160–61, 162
   UPFs and, 223
microdosing, 276
microtransactions, 257–58
middle childhood
   ages and stages in, 25–33. *See also* ages and stages in middle childhood
   author's story, 6–7
   changes in, 34–35
   developmental theories of, 22–25, 34–35
   as "forgotten years," 4, 6, 7–8, 20, 287
   gender identity, 180
   key milestones of, 21
   Nora's story, 1, 2–4
   overlooking of, 1–2, 8–9
   overview of, 7–9
   parental role, 4–5, 13–15, 19–44. *See also* parental role
   use of term, 8
milk glands, 74
mindful eating, 230
mindfulness, 9, 98–102, 132–35, 138
   breathing, 99–100, 132–33
   mantras, 101, 134
   nature immersion, 133–34
   yoga, meditation, and movement, 101, 134–35
minimally processed foods, 223–24
mirror checking, 191–92, 193
misattunement, 105
modeling
   abstinence and drinking, 281, 285
   consent, 188
   eating, 218
   emotional intelligence, 145
   emotional regulation, 98, 102, 115, 116–17, 131
   empathy and kindness, 151, 152
   positive self-talk, 201
   "tear and repair," 102–3
monotasking, 101–2
mood changes, 81–82
moral development
   age six, 26
   age seven, 27
   age eight, 29
   age nine, 30
   age ten, 31
   ages eleven and twelve, 32

movement, 135. *See also* dancing; exercise; sports
multitasking, 101–2
Murthy, Vivek, 10, 234, 244

National Education Association (NEA), 149
National Institute of Mental Health (NIMH), 212, 215–16
National Institutes of Health (NIH), 8, 219, 223
nature immersion, 133–34
nature vs. nurture, 180–81
neglectful parenting style, 41–42
Netflix, 234, 262
neuroplasticity, 91–92, 99
new rules of puberty, 45–84
   Ava and Carolyn's story, 45–46, 49
   development of the body. *See* body development
   FAQs, 52–55
   race and, 48, 60–62
   "The Talk." *See* "Talk, The"
nicotine, 236, 281–83
nicotine pouches, 283–84
nocturnal emissions, 54, 71–72
nonbiological, 82
nonconformity. *See* gender nonconformity
nonverbal processing, 105, 121

obesity. *See* childhood obesity
obsessive-compulsive disorder (OCD), 9, 192, 206, 213
omega-3 fatty acids, 243
online business models, 262–63
online gambling, 258–59
online grooming, 252–53
online privacy, 250, 252
online screen use. *See* screen time
online sources, reliable/unreliable, 251–52
OpenAI, 253
opioids, 3, 271
outbursts, 89, 90, 98, 100, 116. *See also* anger
   the Volcano, 126–27
ovaries, 52, 57, 63–65, 75, 76, 81
overachievers, 144

Palihapitiya, Chamath, 241
panic attacks, 10–11, 154
pansexual, 165
paradigm shifts, 5–6, 14, 22
   body image, 196–97
   emotional changes, 91, 119
   pressure, 143

puberty, 51
screen time, 238
sexual and gender identity, 167
parasympathetic nervous system, 99
parental controls, 210, 246, 247, 269
parental pressure and perfectionism, 140–43
parental role, 4–5, 13–15, 19–44
   ages and stages in middle childhood and, 25–33
   developing competency, 35–37
   emotional regulation and. *See* emotional regulation and parents
   Hannah and Chris's story, 19–20, 21, 35, 37–38, 42–43, 44
   school pressure and perfectionism, 140–43
   stages of active parenting, 33–34
parenting books, 7–8
parenting styles, 37–43
   authoritarian, 39–40, 42
   authoritative, 38–39, 42
   permissive, 40–41, 42
   uninvolved/neglectful, 41–42
parent time-outs, 116–17
passwords, smartphone, 246
peer pressure, 4, 30–31, 199, 276, 282
penises, 46–47, 54, 57, 63–64, 70–71, 168
perfectionism, 140–42
period. *See* menstruation
"period pouches," 80
permissive parenting style, 40–41, 42
phones. *See* apps; screen time; smartphones
physical bullying, 148
Piaget, Jean, 23
picky eaters, 216, 217–18
pituitary glands, 52
plastic surgery, 207, 266
Plato, 87
play, 26, 43, 168
   importance of, 43–44
   school pressure and, 145, 163
playdates, 21, 34, 35, 237
pornography, 177–78, 188
positive reinforcement, 29, 31, 200–201. *See also* praise
   affirmations, 134
positive self-talk, 27, 201
poverty, 61, 219
praise (praising), 29, 36, 42, 95, 141, 145, 163, 200–201, 218
prefrontal cortexes, 49, 91, 132, 235
prejudicial bullying, 148–49

pressure, 3, 11, 139–63. *See also* school pressure
   Cici's story, 139–43
   paradigm shift, 143
   sports and, 158–62
privacy, 88–89, 120, 166
   online, 250, 252
   puberty and, 51, 71, 72
proactive planning, 123–25
problem-solving, 36–37, 43, 115, 152
   age six, 26
   age seven, 27
   age eight, 28
   age nine, 30
   age ten, 31
   ages eleven and twelve, 32
processed foods, 48, 222–24, 230
procrastination, 140. *See also* avoidance
psilocybin mushrooms, 276
"psychological invalidation," 108–9
psychologists, shortage in, 12–13
psychosexual development, 22–23
PTSD (post-traumatic stress disorder), 6, 276
puberty
   age, 47–50, 52, 53
   for boys, 2, 49–50, 52–53, 54–55, 59–60, 64–65
   brain development, 49, 52, 54–55
   coping strategies for, 83–84
   developmental stages, 22–23
   early onset. *See* earlier puberty
   FAQs, 52–55
   gender differences, 2, 49–50, 52–53
   for girls, 2, 49–50, 52–55, 63–64
   middle childhood overlap, 37
   new rules of. *See* new rules of puberty
   Nora's story, 1, 2–4
   paradigm shift, 5–6, 51
   parental comfort talking about, 45–47, 50–51, 55–60
   race and, 60–62
   signs of, 51–52
   use of term, 48
pubic hair, 52, 69–70
purging, 199, 212

race
   childhood obesity and, 219
   earlier puberty and, 48, 60–62
   mental health care, 13, 61
   prejudicial bullying, 148–49
race-to-college mindset, 146–47
reactive parenting, 110–11, 221

reframing, 14, 125–26. *See also* paradigm shifts
relational bullying, 148
reliable/unreliable sources, 251–52
replacement behaviors, 125–26, 193
reproductive systems
   of boys, 70–72
   of girls, 59, 75, 76, 77–78
responsibilities
   age six, 27
   age seven, 28
   age eight, 29
   age nine, 30
   age ten, 31
   ages eleven and twelve, 33
responsive parenting, 110–11
restrictive diet, 199, 202, 211, 212, 214–15, 216, 226
Roblox, 233, 259
Robux, 259
Roe v. Wade, 11
role models, 183, 211, 229, 268
role playing, 124–25
rumination, 92, 133–34

sadness, 9, 10, 119, 173, 182, 234
schedules (scheduling), 141, 145
schools, 139–63
   bullying in, 147–52. *See also* bullying
   parents and attunement, 106
   sex education, 47, 49, 58, 72, 164, 165, 167
   social-emotional learning, 121–22
school absenteeism, 149, 154, 156
   Alex's story, 152–53
school anxiety, 152–58, 167. *See also* school pressure
   active shooter drills, 3, 157–58
   Alex's story, 152–53
   avoidance and, 140, 152–58
   Cici's story, 139–41
   dos and dont's, 155–56
   Jay's story, 158–59
   Nora's story, 2–4
   perfectionism and parental pressure, 140–42
school grades, 141, 146, 154
school pressure, 143–52. *See also* bullying
   Cici's story, 139–43
   parents and, 140–43
   race-to-college mindset, 146–47
   sports and, 158–62
school refusal, 152–58
   Alex's story, 152–53
   effects of, 154
school shootings, 3, 157
   active shooter drills, 3, 157–58

screen-free zones, 232–33, 237–38, 239, 245, 246–48, 252, 268
screen time, 48, 182, 231–69
   ADHD and, 242–43
   brain development and, 235–36, 243, 260–61
   digital citizenship, 248–50
   digital detox, 267–68
   dopamine and, 240–42
   harms of, 233–37, 238
   Jon's story, 231–33, 237
   paradigm shift, 238
   parents and multitasking, 102
   red flags, 238–39
   setting limits, 232–35, 237–38, 239, 245, 246–48, 252, 268–69
   sleep and, 239–40
   Wait Until 8th pledge, 244, 245, 269
scrotum, 66, 70
search engines, 253
self-compassion, 30, 151, 182, 201
self-efficacy, 35–37
self-esteem
   age six, 26
   age seven, 27
   age eight, 28
   age nine, 29
   age ten, 31
   ages eleven and twelve, 32
   body image connection, 199–201, 202
   building up, 200–201
   parenting styles and, 40, 41
   thought replacements, 125–26
self-expression, 145
   age six, 26
   age seven, 28
   age eight, 29
   age nine, 30
   age ten, 31
   ages eleven and twelve, 33
self-fulfilling prophecies, 125–26
self-regulation, 92, 96–98, 137–38. *See also* emotional regulation
self-soothing, 183
sense of control, 74, 92, 117, 123, 131–32
sense of self, 35
sex education, 47, 49, 58, 72, 164, 165, 167
sex talk. *See* "Talk, The"
"sextortion," 252
sexual abuse, 47, 149, 182
sexual bullying, 148
sexual consent, 174–75, 177, 188

Index

sexual development, 45–47, 49–50, 55
  boys' reproductive system, 70–72
  girls' breast development, 73–74
  girls' reproductive system, 75, 76, 77–78
  masturbation, 71, 72
  menstruation, 80–83
  parental comfort talking about, 45–47, 50–51, 55–60, 62–65, 175–78. *See also* "Talk, The"
  sexual identities and, 168–70
sexual identity, 3–4, 14, 164–78
  age-appropriate talk about sex, 175–78
  author's story, 164–65
  development, 168–70
  gender identity vs., 178–79
  LGBTQ+, 170–74
  paradigm shift, 167
  signs and red flags, 167
  understanding relationships and consent, 174–75
sexually transmitted diseases, 175–76, 177
sexual orientation, 169–72
shame (shaming), 29, 88, 112
  body shaming, 203–5
  puberty and, 46, 47, 50, 55, 83
shaving, 69–70
siblings, 36–37, 106, 129–30, 166, 174–75
Siegel, Dan, 93
Sinek, Simon, 231
skin care, 78
sleep, 88. *See also* bedtime
  screen time before, 239–40
sleepovers, 164, 177, 203, 227, 237
smartphones. *See also* apps; screen time
  ADHD and, 242–43
  guide to giving child first, 245–48
  harms of, 233–37, 238
  setting limits, 232–35, 237–38, 239, 245, 246–48, 252, 268–69
  sleep and, 239–40
  Wait Until 8th pledge, 244, 245, 269
smoking, 236, 281–83
Snapchat, 263
social constructs, 180–83
  for boys, 181–83
  for girls, 182–83
social-emotional learning, 35, 121–22
  age six, 25–26
  age seven, 27
  age eight, 28
  age nine, 29
  age ten, 30–31
  ages eleven and twelve, 32
social hierarchies, 30–31, 148

social media, 3, 9, 259–61
  algorithms, 261–62, 272
  beauty culture, 265–66
  body image and, 194, 198–99
  brain development and screen time, 235–36, 243, 260–61
  dopamine and, 240–42
  harms, 259–60
  harms of, 233–37, 238
  influencers, 264–66
  online business models, 262–63
social pressure. *See* pressure; school pressure
"solution seekers," 124–25
somatosensory cortex, 236
sore breasts, 81–82
sperm, 52, 57, 63–65
spiraling tornado, 129–30
sports, 2, 158–62, 196
  benefits of, 160–62
  discontinuation of, 159–60
  Jay's story, 158–59
Start with the Talk, 7, 164–66
stereotypes, 148–49, 181, 210
  gender, 181–82, 210
Stop, Breathe, Think, Then Act ("Stop and Think"), 130–31, 137
stress, 2, 3, 21, 48, 88, 118, 139, 235. *See also* pressure; school anxiety; school pressure
  alcohol and, 280–81
  body awareness for, 135–37
  body image and food, 208, 209, 213, 214, 217, 227–28
  digital detox for, 267–68
  maternal, 220, 243
  mindfulness for, 99–102, 132–35
  PTSD, 6, 276
  race and, 61–62
  school refusal, 152–58
stretching, 135
structure, 4, 94–95
substance abuse, 270–85
  alcohol, 278–81
  earlier puberty in girls and, 48
  Emilia and Celeste's story, 270–73
  gender dysphoria and, 187
  global youth mental health crisis, 10
  marijuana, 273–77
  nicotine, 281–83
  obesity and, 219
  permissive parental style and, 41
sugar, 224–25, 230

suicide (suicidal ideation), 12–13
    BDD and, 206, 207
    gender dysphoria and, 187
    incidence of, 11
    LGBTQ+ children, 13, 173–74
    social media use and, 235
    team sport participation for reducing risk, 160–61
summer enrichment programs, 146–47
sweating. *See* body odor
sympathetic nervous system, 99
synaptic pruning, 54

"Talk, The," 55–60, 175–78
    getting mentally prepared for, 56–57
    parental comfort about, 45–47, 50–51, 55–60
    questions from children, 65–66
    sample scripts, 58–60
    setting an intention, 56–57
    sex scripts for children, 62–65
    topics to cover, 176–77
    top 10 tips for, 57–58
tantrums, 10, 111, 117, 118, 154
"tear and repair," 102–3
teeth
    baby, and Tooth Fairy, 24–25
    body image and, 207, 210
    brushing, 56, 93
    grinding (bruxism), 136
    whitening, 207
testicles (testes), 52, 54, 57, 63, 64, 70, 168
testosterone, 52, 70–71, 78, 181
THC (tetrahydrocannabinol), 272, 274–75
thought replacements, 125–26, 138
TikTok, 78, 195, 233, 234, 272
time-outs, 89, 112, 130
    Stop, Breathe, Think, Then Act, 130–31, 137
tomboys, 179
Tooth Fairy, 24–25
Tornado, the, 129–30
toys, 44, 83, 181, 183, 210
transgender, 170, 173, 186
Trevor Project, 173
triggers
    attunement, 104–7
    identifying, 123–25
    Leila's story, 193
    Stop, Breathe, Think, Then Act, 130–31, 137

    the Volcano, 126–27
    window of tolerance, 93–96
Twenge, Jean, 234–35

ultra-processed foods (UPFs), 222–24, 230
underage drinking, 278–81
underarm hair, 52, 69–70
uninvolved parenting style, 41–42
University of North Carolina, 259–60
uterus, 57, 64, 75, 76, 77

vacations, 192, 194, 203, 232–33, 237
vagina, 53, 57, 63–64, 76, 77–78
vaginal discharge, 77–78
validation, 108–10, 174, 207
vaping, 281–83
verbal bullying, 148
video games, 123, 142, 236–37, 255–57. *See also* screen time
    ADHD and, 242–143
    creating safety and boundaries, 256–57
    dopamine and, 240–42
    Jon's story, 231–33, 237
    microtransactions, 257–58
    ratings of, 257
visual metaphors, 126–30
    the Iceberg, 128–29
    the Tornado, 129–30
    the Volcano, 126–27, 127
vocal folds, 73
voice changes, 73
Volcano, the, 126–27, 127
vulva, 47, 77

Wait Until 8th pledge, 244, 245, 269
waxing hair, 69
weight changes, 66–67
weight loss, 213, 225–26, 261
wet dreams, 54, 71–72
What's Happening to Me? (Meredith), 46
"Who holds the energy here?", 104
whole foods, 223
window of tolerance, 93–96, 95
working memory, 92, 235
worry, 11, 154, 155–56, 195

yoga, 100–101, 134–35
Yoga Pretzels, 134–35
YouTube, 135, 231, 233, 234, 239, 242, 244, 262

ZYN, 283–84

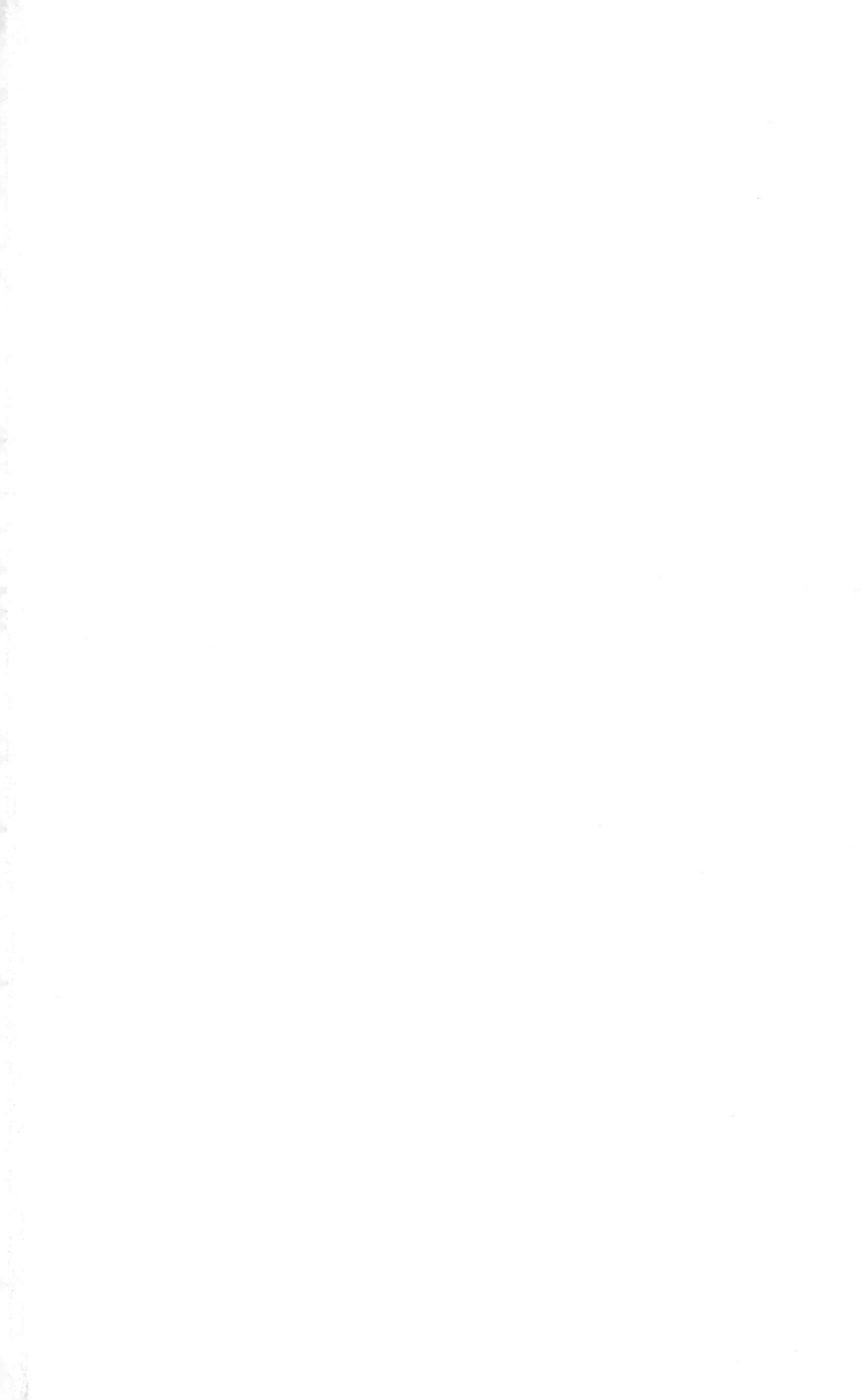